Curing IBS Naturally

with Chinese Medicine

Jane Bean

BLUE POPPY PRESS

Published by:

BLUE POPPY PRESS
A Division of Blue Poppy Enterprises, Inc.
5441 Western Ave., #2
BOULDER, CO 80301

First Edition, September, 1999
Second Printing, July 2000
Third Printing, January, 2002
Fourth Printing, April, 2003
Fifth Printing, March, 2004
Sixth Printing, February, 2005
Seventh Printing, February, 2006
Eighth Printing, September, 2007
Ninth Printing, January, 2009

ISBN 1-891845-11-X
IASBN 978-1-891845-11-X
LC# 99-72726

The information in this book is given in good faith. However, the translators and the publishers cannot be held responsible for any error or omission. Nor can they be held in any way responsible for treatment given on the basis of information contained in this book. The publishers make this information available to English language readers for scholarly and research purposes only.

The publishers do not advocate nor endorse self-medication by laypersons. Chinese medicine is a professional medicine. Laypersons interested in availing themselves of the treatments described in this book should seek out a qualified professional practitioner of Chinese medicine.

COMP Designation: Original work
Cover design by Eric Brearton
Printed at Fidlar Doubleday, Kalamazoo, MI

10 9

Other books in this series include:

Curing Insomnia Naturally with Chinese Medicine
Curing Hay Fever Naturally with Chinese Medicine
Curing Headaches Naturally with Chinese Medicine
Better Breast Health Naturally with Chinese Medicine
Curing Depression Naturally with Chinese Medicine
Curing Arthritis Naturally with Chinese Medicine
Curing PMS Naturally with Chinese Medicine
Managing Menopause Naturally with Chinese Medicine
Curing Fibromyalgia Naturally with Chinese Medicine
Controlling Diabetes Naturally with Chinese Medicine

Preface

I began my study of traditional Chinese medicine 12 years ago. In my classes at acupuncture school, as we studied various diseases, we would go over the Chinese causes of disease over and over again. These were always something like improper eating, too much work, too much emotional upset, not enough exercise, or not enough rest. I remember thinking that these were repetitive and rather simplistic ideas.

Now, having been in practice for eight years and having experienced both the effectiveness of Chinese medicine and the cohesiveness of its system of thought, I know that these ideas are not simplistic, but rather simple. They are also very powerful. I have come to see that these simple things that cause ill health according to the theory of traditional Chinese medicine are truly the cause of most disease. They are, by and large, also all within our personal power to control.

Therefore, in this book on irritable bowel syndrome (IBS), we will look at how IBS is diagnosed and treated in general by traditional Chinese medicine. We will then go on to discuss treatment by professional practitioners as well as numerous safe, no or low cost, and effective self-treatments. In Chinese medicine, it is said that the superior doctor is one who prevents disease. Such prevention is done by educating the patient. By writing this book on the diagnosis and treatment of IBS with Chinese medicine, I hope I have continued this tradition by giving those with this disorder the tools they need to help keep themselves healthy.

Thanks are due to Bob Flaws for his generous use of materials from other Blue Poppy *Curing* books and for his help in preparing this book.

Jane Bean
Brattleboro, VT
April, 1999

Table of Contents

1 Introduction

Rosemary had suffered from irritable bowel syndrome for most of her adult life, but in the past few months the symptoms had gotten a lot worse. Even though she had severely limited her diet to try to prevent the attacks of cramping and diarrhea, on a bad day, she had to make at least five or six trips to the bathroom. It was embarrassing to have to interrupt meetings with clients, and, if she needed to take someone to lunch, she had to make sure they went to a restaurant where she had checked out the location of the bathroom beforehand. Her symptoms were creating an added stress in her life that was making her feel more and more tired.

Jim was the kind of guy who worked hard and played hard. Except for a few sports injuries, he considered himself pretty healthy. Years ago, a doctor had told him that he had a nervous stomach, and he had learned to live with it. Sometimes he had constipation and sometimes diarrhea. Often he had bloating or cramping with the urge to go to the bathroom, but, when he got there, nothing would happen. If he could go, he would feel better. Most of the time, Jim ate sensibly, but occasionally, he would treat himself to premium ice cream or a cup of coffee, even though he knew he would pay for it later.

Sound familiar? If so, this book may very well help you break the cycle of IBS. According to traditional Chinese medicine, irritable bowel syndrome is most definitely classified as a valid gastrointestinal complaint or disease. The good news is that Chinese doctors (including acupuncturists) have been curing IBS for centuries if not millennia.

This book is a layperson's guide to the diagnosis and treatment of IBS with Chinese medicine. In it, you will learn what causes IBS *and what you can do about it.* Hopefully, you will be able to identify yourself and your symptoms in these pages. If you can see yourself in the signs and symptoms discussed below, you will be able to choose from a number of self-help techniques the ones which will help you. Chinese medicine cannot cure every gastrointestinal disease, but, when it comes to IBS, Chinese medicine is one of the best alternatives I know. When someone calls and says that IBS is their main complaint, I know that, if they follow my advice, together we can cure, or at least reduce, the signs and symptoms of their irritable bowel.

What is IBS?

The Merck Manual defines irritable bowel syndrome (also known as spastic colon or mucous colitis) as "motility disorders involving the small intestine and large bowel associated with variable degrees of abdominal pain, constipation, or diarrhea, largely as a reaction to stress in a susceptible individual."[1] The abdominal pain tends to be triggered by eating and may be relieved after a bowel movement. It may be accompanied by other gastrointestinal complaints, such as bloating, flatulence, nausea, passage of mucous, a feeling of incomplete emptying, or pain in the anus and rectum. IBS also has a range of symptoms that are not digestive in nature. Among these are headache, fatigue, lassitude, depression, anxiety, and poor concentration. Luckily, any given person with IBS will not experience all these symptoms. Most people tend to experience a few of them, usually pretty much the same ones, periodically.

Is IBS really a disease?

IBS is one of the purely *functional* gastrointestinal disorders. Although this disorder has always existed, it was not recognized by Western medicine until about 50 years ago and has only become a common diagnosis in the last 20 years. By definition in

[1] *The Merck Manual of Diagnosis and Therapy*, Robert Berkow, MD, editor, Merck, Sharp, and Dohme Research Laboratories, Rahway, NJ, 1987, p. 808

Western medical theory, a functional disorder is one where there is *no* known structural (meaning anatomical), biochemical, or infectious cause. When such a disorder presents as a group of symptoms which tend to occur together it is called a "syndrome." Looking at irritability of the bowel as a syndrome allows MDs to recognize this condition as a clinical entity and to develop and prescribe treatments for it.

The symptoms of IBS are similar to those of other common diseases, some of which can be quite serious. Conditions that may be confused with IBS include lactose intolerance, bacterial or parasitic infection, and colon or ovarian cancers, to name just a few. For this reason, depending on the severity of a person's symptoms, their age, and their general health, testing may be required to rule out other possible conditions before a diagnosis of IBS is reached.

It is estimated that 10-20% of all American adults experience symptoms of IBS. Even though only half of these visit a doctor, patients with IBS account for one-half of all gastrointestinal (GI) referrals or initial visits for GI complaints. IBS affects three times as many women as men, and, after the common cold, is the next most common cause of missed school and work.[2]

What causes IBS?

The symptoms of IBS are caused by abnormal motility (or movement) and increased pain sensitivity of the gut. Motor function may be lower than normal, causing diarrhea. Increased frequency and strength of contractions in the colon cause constipation. Pain is caused both by increased contractions or spasms and by heightened sensitivity of the nerves in the intestinal tract. People with IBS may experience pain even from normal contractions and normal amounts of intestinal gas.

---

[2] http://www.broadwing.medunc.edu/medicine/fgidc, UNC Functional Gastro-intestinal Disorders Center, Douglas A. Drossman, MD, and William E. Whitehead, MD, co-directors.

Both initial and subsequent episodes of IBS can be triggered by emotional factors, foods, some medicines, and hormones. Many people with IBS have a history of either parasitic infections or early trauma, including physical or sexual abuse.

No one knows why some people develop heightened sensitivity of the GI tract, at least in terms of Western medicine, but researchers are working on the theory that there are direct links between the GI tract and the central nervous system. Such a brain-gut connection would explain why emotional upsets affect the intestines and why intestinal symptoms affect mood. In addition, in an effort to more completely understand irritability of the bowel, researchers are developing more sophisticated and sensitive techniques to measure physiological activity in the gastrointestinal tract.

How Western medicine treats IBS

When Western MDs try to treat IBS, they usually do so using a combination of diet and lifestyle changes coupled with a prescription for one or more Western pharmaceuticals which are used as needed to treat the symptoms of constipation, diarrhea, pain, and mental-emotional discomfort. For constipation, a fiber supplement, such as bran or psyllium seeds, is recommended to increase the diameter of the colon and reduce the pressure inside. This takes 1-2 months to work. So medication may be prescribed on a temporary basis to relieve spastic pain. An anticholinergic agent, alone or in combination with a mild tranquilizer or sedative, may be used for this purpose. Diarrhea is treated with medications that slow peristalsis and reduce intestinal spasm. Tranquilizers and antidepressants are used to deal with nervousness, anxiety, and depression.

Unfortunately, many people experience side effects from any or all of these types of Western medication. Propantheline, the anticholinergic agent suggested by the authors of *The Merck Manual* for treating spastic pain accompanying constipation, may actually cause constipation as well as difficulty in urination, skin rash or hives, headache, eye pain, sensitivity to light, blurred vision, nausea, vomiting, dry mouth, loss of taste, flushing, fever, drowsiness, weakness, and sleeplessness.[3] Loperamide (Immodium) and diphenoxylate (Lomotil) may be used to treat diarrhea. The most common side effect of Immodium is constipation. Occasionally, it may cause nausea, abdominal pain, dizziness, or dry mouth.[4] Likewise, Lomotil commonly causes gastrointestinal symptoms such as nausea, vomiting, and abdominal distention and may cause other side effects, such as drowsiness, dizziness, numbness of the extremities, blurred vision, weakness, and mental depression. Symptoms of over-dosage with this medication, which may not show up for 24-30 hours after it is taken, include tachycardia, dry nose, throat and mouth, flushing, and fever.[5] Amitriptyline, more commonly known as Elavil, is the cyclic antidepressant *The Merck Manual* recommends for IBS, in low doses for its anticholinergic effects and often in higher doses for depression. The *AARP Prescription Drug Handbook* lists over 60 possible side effects for Elavil. Of particular relevance to those with IBS is that Elavil can cause either constipation or diarrhea.[6] Thus, many people cannot take or do not want to take these types of Western pharmaceuticals.

Happily, many Western clinicians recognize that diet and lifestyle play a part in the cause, treatment, and prevention of IBS. In terms of diet, Western MDs typically make recommendations based on symptoms. When abdominal distention and flatulence are a problem, typically MDs advise

---

3 *AARP Pharmacy Service Prescription Drug Handbook,* second edition,Nancy J. Olins, MA, senior editor, Harper Collins Publishers, Inc., New York, NY, 1992, pp. 382-385

4 Clayton, Bruce D., *Mosby's Handbook of Pharmacology*, fourth edition, The C. V. Mosby Company, St. Louis, MO, 1987, p. 721

5 *Ibid.* p. 711

6 *AARP Prescription Drug Handbook, op. cit.*, pp. 622-623

reducing or eliminating beans, cabbage, and other foods high in fermentable carbohydrates, such as fruit juices and dried fruits. A low fat diet with increased protein is recommended for those who have abdominal pain after eating. Bland bulking agents, such as the bran and psyllium previously mentioned, are suggested for those with constipation, and those with lactose intolerance are obviously advised to avoid dairy products. Basically, Chinese doctors agree with these dietary recommendations but make even more precise and extensive ones, fine tuning each person's diet to uniquely fit them.

In terms of lifestyle, many Western clinicians today are aware of the mind-body connection that plays such a large role in IBS. Therefore, they may recommend some form of stress reduction, counseling, or possibly psychotherapy. Regular exercise is often recommended to reduce stress and to normalize bowel function in those who are constipated. Later on, we will also talk about these from the Chinese point of view.

However, although proper diet and lifestyle are necessary to keep the symptoms of IBS from recurring, they may not be sufficient by themselves to eliminate the symptoms that are already present. Therefore, for many people, dietary changes, counseling, and stress reduction are not enough.

Western medicine, by its own admission, has no cure for IBS.[7] The best it has to offer at the present time is a collection of treatments meant to alleviate the symptoms of IBS. Happily, since Chinese medicine does cure IBS *without side effects*, it does offer a safe and effective alternative to the types of pharmaceuticals discussed above.

7 *The Merck Manual, op. cit.* p. 810

East is East and West is West

In order for the reader to understand and make sense of the rest of this book on Chinese medicine and IBS, one must understand that Chinese medicine is a distinct and separate system of medical thought and practice from modern Western medicine. This means that one must shift models of reality when it comes to thinking about Chinese medicine. It has taken the Chinese more than 2,000 years to develop this medical system. In fact, Chinese medicine is the oldest continually practiced, literate, professional medicine in the world. As such one cannot understand Chinese medicine by trying to explain it in Western scientific or medical terms.

Most people reading this book have probably taken high school biology back when they were sophomores. Whether we recognize it or not, most of us Westerners think of what we learned about the human body in high school as "the really real" description of reality, not one possible description. However, if Chinese medicine is to make any sense to Westerners at all, one must be able to entertain the notion that there are potentially other valid descriptions of the human body, its functions, health, and disease. In grappling with this fundamentally important issue, it is useful to think about the concepts of a map and the terrain it describes.

If we take the United States of America as an example, we can have numerous different maps of this country's land mass. One map might show population. Another might show per capita incomes. Another might show religious or ethnic distributions. Yet another might be a road map. And still another might be a map showing political, *i.e.*, state boundaries. In fact, there could be an infinite number of potentially different maps of the United States depending on what one was trying to show and do. As long as the map is based on accurate information and has been created with self-consistent logic, then one map is not necessarily more correct than another. The issue is to use the right map for what you are trying to do. If one wants to drive from Chicago to Washington, DC, then a road map is probably the right one *for that job* but is not necessarily a truer or "more real" description of the United States than a map showing annual rainfall.

What I am getting at here is that *the map is not the terrain.* The Western biological map of the human body is only one potentially useful medical map. It is no more true than the traditional Chinese medical map, and the "facts" of one map cannot be reduced to the criteria or standards of another *unless they share the same logic right from the beginning.* As long as the Western medical map is capable of solving a person's disease in a cost-effective, time-efficient manner without side effects or iatrogenesis (meaning doctor-caused disease), then it is a useful map. Chinese medicine needs to be judged in the same way. The Chinese medical map of health and disease is just as "real" as the Western biological map as long as by using it professional practitioners are able to solve their patients' health problems in a safe and effective way.

Therefore, the following chapter is an introduction to the basics of Chinese medicine. Unless one understands some of the fundamental theories and "facts" of Chinese medicine, one will not be able to understand or accept the reasons for some of the Chinese medical treatments of IBS. As the reader will quickly see from this brief overview of Chinese medicine, "This doesn't look like Kansas, Toto!"

2
An Overview of the Chinese Medical Map

In this chapter, we will look at an overview of Chinese medicine. In particular, we will discuss yin and yang, qi, blood, and essence, the viscera and bowels, and the channels and network vessels. Then, in the following chapter, we will go on to see how Chinese medicine views the disease mechanisms that cause IBS. After that, we will look at the Chinese medical diagnosis and treatment of the symptoms of IBS.

Yin & Yang

To understand Chinese medicine, one must first understand the concepts of yin and yang since these are the most basic concepts in this system. Yin and yang are the cornerstones for understanding, diagnosing, and treating the body and mind in Chinese medicine. In a sense, all the other theories and concepts of Chinese medicine are nothing other than an elaboration of yin and yang. Most people have probably already heard of yin and yang but may have only a fuzzy idea of what these terms mean.

The concepts of yin and yang can be used to describe everything that exists in the universe, including all the parts and functions of the body. Originally, yin referred to the shady side of a hill and yang to the sunny side of the hill. Since sunshine and shade are two, interdependent sides of a single reality, these two aspects of the hill are seen as part of a single whole. Other examples of yin and yang are that night exists only in relation to day and cold exists only in relation to heat. According to Chinese thought, every single thing that exists in the universe has these two aspects, a yin and a yang. Thus everything has a front and a back, a top and a bottom, a left and a right, and a beginning and an end. However, a thing is yin or yang *only in relation to its paired complement.* Nothing is in itself yin or yang.

It is the concepts of yin and yang which make Chinese medicine a holistic medicine. This is because, based on this unitary and complementary vision of reality, no body part or body function is viewed as separate or isolated from the whole person. The table below shows a partial list of yin and yang pairs as they apply to the body.

Yin	Yang
form	function
organs	bowels
blood	qi
inside	outside
front of body	back of body
right side	left side
lower body	upper body
cool, cold	warm, hot
stillness	activity, movement

However, it is important to remember that each item listed is either yin or yang only in relation to its complementary partner. Nothing is absolutely and all by itself either yin or yang. As we can see from the above list, it is possible to describe every aspect of the body in terms of yin and yang.

Qi

Qi (pronounced chee) and blood are the two most important complementary pairs of yin and yang within the human body. It is said that, in the world, yin and yang are water and fire, but in the human body, yin and yang are blood and qi. Qi is yang in relation to blood which is yin. Qi is often translated as energy and certainly energy is a manifestation of qi. Chinese language scholars would say, however, that qi is larger than any single type of energy described by modern Western science. Paul Unschuld, perhaps the greatest living sinologist, translates the word qi as influences. This conveys the sense that qi is what is responsible for change and movement. Thus, within Chinese medicine, qi is that which motivates all movement and transformation or change.

In Chinese medicine, qi is defined as having five specific functions:

1. Defense

It is qi which is responsible for protecting the exterior of the body from invasion by external pathogens. This qi, called defensive qi, flows through the exterior portion of the body.

2. Transformation

Qi transforms substances so that they can be utilized by the body. An example of this function is the transformation of the food we eat into nutrients to nourish the body, thus producing more qi and blood.

3. Warming

Qi, being relatively yang, is inherently warm and one of the main functions of the qi is to warm the entire body, both inside and out. If this warming function of the qi is weak, cold may cause the flow of qi and blood to be congealed similar to cold's effect on water producing ice.

4. Restraint

It is qi which holds all the organs and substances in their proper place. Thus all the organs, blood, and fluids need qi to keep them from falling or leaking out of their specific pathways. If this function of the qi is weak, then problems like uterine prolapse, easy bruising, or urinary incontinence may occur.

5. Transportation

Qi provides the motivating force for all transportation and movement in the body. Every aspect of the body that moves is moved by the qi. Hence the qi moves the blood and body fluids throughout the body. It moves food through the stomach and blood through the vessels.

Blood

In Chinese medicine, blood refers to the red fluid that flows through our vessels the same as in modern Western medicine, but it also has meanings and implications which are different from those in modern Western medicine. Most basically, blood is that substance which nourishes and moistens all the body tissues. Without blood, no body tissue can function properly. In addition, when blood is insufficient or scanty, tissue becomes dry and withers.

Qi and blood are closely interrelated. It is said that, "Qi is the commander of the blood and blood is the mother of qi." This means that it is qi which moves the blood but that it is the blood which provides the nourishment and physical foundation for the creation and existence of the qi.

In Chinese medicine, blood provides the following functions for the body:

1. Nourishment

Blood nourishes the body. Along with qi, the blood goes to every part of the body. When the blood is insufficient, function decreases and tissue atrophies or shrinks.

2. Moistening

Blood moistens the body tissues. This includes the skin, eyes, and ligaments and tendons or what are simply called the sinews of the body in Chinese medicine. Thus blood insufficiency can cause drying out and consequent stiffening of various body tissues throughout the body.

3. Blood provides the material foundation for the spirit or mind.

In Chinese medicine, the mind and body are not two separate things. The spirit is nothing other than a great accumulation of qi. The blood (yin) supplies the material support and nourishment for the spirit (yang) so that it accumulates, becomes bright (*i.e.*, conscious and clever), and stays rooted in the body. If the blood becomes insufficient, the mind can "float," causing problems like insomnia, agitation, and unrest.

Essence

Along with qi and blood, essence is one of the three most important constituents of the body. Essence is the most fundamental, essential material the body utilizes for its growth, maturation, and reproduction. There are two forms of this essence. We inherit essence from our parents and we also produce our own essence from the food we eat, the liquids we drink, and the air we breathe.

The essence which comes from our parents is what determines our basic constitution, strength, and vitality. We each have a finite, limited amount of this inherited essence. It is important to protect and conserve this essence because all bodily functions depend upon it, and, when it is gone, we die. Thus the depletion of essence has serious implications for our overall health and well-being. Happily, the essence derived from food and drink helps to bolster and support this inherited essence. Thus, if we eat well and do not consume more qi and blood than we create each day, then when we sleep at night, this surplus qi and more especially blood is transformed into essence.

The Viscera & Bowels

In Chinese medicine, the internal organs (called viscera so as not to become confused with the Western biological entities of the same name) have a wider area of function and influence than in Western medicine. Each viscus has distinct responsibilities for maintaining the physical and psychological health of the individual. When thinking about the internal viscera according to Chinese medicine, it is more accurate to view them as spheres of influence or a network that spreads throughout the body, rather than as a distinct and separate physical organ as described by Western science. This is why the famous German sinologist, Manfred Porkert, refers to them as orbs rather than as organs. In Chinese medicine, the relationship between the various viscera and other parts of the body is made possible by the channel and network vessel system which we will discuss below.

In Chinese medicine, there are five main viscera which are relatively yin and six main bowels which are relatively yang. The five yin viscera are the heart, lungs, liver, spleen, and kidneys. The six yang bowels are the stomach, small intestine, large intestine, gallbladder, urinary bladder, and a system that Chinese medicine refers to as the triple burner. All the functions of the entire body are subsumed or described under these eleven organs or spheres of influence. Thus Chinese medicine *as a system* does not have a pancreas, a pituitary gland, or the ovaries. Nonetheless, all the functions of these Western organs are described under the Chinese medical system of the five viscera and six bowels.

Within this system, the five viscera are the most important. These are the organs that Chinese medicine says are responsible for the creation and transformation of qi and blood and the storage of essence. For instance, the kidneys are responsible for the excretion of urine but are also responsible for hearing, the strength of the bones, sex, reproduction, maturation and growth, the lower and upper back, and the lower legs in general and the knees in particular.

Visceral Correspondences

Organ	Tissue	Sense	Spirit	Emotion
Kidneys	bones/ head hair	hearing	will	fear
Liver	sinews	sight	ethereal soul	anger
Spleen	flesh	taste	thought	thinking/ worry
Lungs	skin/body hair	smell	corporeal soul	grief/ sadness
Heart	blood vessels	speech	spirit	joy/fright

This points out that the Chinese viscera may have the same name and even some overlapping functions but yet are quite different from the organs of modern Western medicine. Each of the five Chinese medical viscera also has a corresponding tissue, sense, spirit, and emotion related to it. These are outlined in the table above.

In addition, each Chinese medical viscus or bowel possesses both a yin and a yang aspect. The yin aspect of a viscus or bowel refers to its substantial nature or tangible form. Further, an organ's yin is responsible for the nurturing, cooling, and moistening of that viscus or bowel. The yang aspect of the viscus or bowel represents its functional activities or what it does. An organ's yang aspect is also warming. These two aspects, yin and yang, form and function, cooling and heating, when balanced create good health. However, if either yin or yang becomes too strong or too weak, the result will be disease.

Below are the key statements of fact about the main viscera and bowels involved in IBS. These are the liver, spleen, kidneys, stomach, and large intestine. The Chinese medical explanation of the cause, mechanisms, diagnosis, and treatment of IBS are all derived from these basic "facts."

The kidneys

In Chinese medicine, the kidneys are considered to be the foundation of our life. Because the developing fetus looks like a large kidney and because the kidneys are the main viscus for the storage of inherited essence, the kidneys are referred to as the prenatal root. Thus keeping the kidney qi strong and kidney yin and yang in relative balance is considered essential to good health and longevity. The basic Chinese medical statements of fact about the kidneys *vis à vis* IBS are:

1. Kidney yin and yang are the foundation for the yin and yang of all the other organs and bowels and body tissues of the entire body.

This is another way of saying that the kidneys are the foundation of our life. If either kidney yin or yang is insufficient, eventually the yin or yang of the other organs will also become insufficient. Vice versa, yin or yang vacuities of the other viscera and bowels may eventually reach kidney yin or yang.

2. The kidneys govern the two yin.

The two yin are the anus and urethra in men and the anus and vaginal opening including the urethra in women. These two orifices are considered "portals" of the kidneys. Therefore, diseases of the large intestine, rectum, and anus are sometimes related to the kidneys.

3. The kidneys govern opening and sealing.

This statement is related to the one above it. It means that the kidneys are responsible for the opening and closing of the anus and urethra. Diarrhea can, therefore, both be due to a kidney qi vacuity and also eventually cause kidney qi vacuity.

4. The low back is the mansion of the kidneys.

Clinically, this means that kidney vacuity is the most common cause of chronic low back. Therefore, low back pain is one of the main symptoms of both kidney yin and kidney yang vacuities.

The liver

In Chinese medicine, the liver is associated with one's emotional state, with digestion, and with menstruation in women. As we will see in the following chapters, the liver plays a major role in the Chinese medical diagnosis and treatment of IBS. The basic Chinese medical statements of facts concerning the liver include:

1. The liver controls coursing and discharge.

Coursing and discharge refer to the uninhibited spreading of qi to every part of the body. If the liver is not able to maintain the free and smooth flow of qi throughout the body, multiple physical and emotional symptoms can develop. This function of the liver is most easily damaged by emotional causes and, in particular, by anger and frustration. For example, if the liver is stressed due to pent-up anger, the flow of liver qi can become depressed or stagnate.

Liver qi stagnation can cause a wide range of health problems, including IBS and other chronic digestive disturbance, premenstrual syndrome, depression, and low back pain. Therefore, it is essential to keep our liver qi flowing freely.

2. The liver stores the blood.

This means that the liver regulates the amount of blood in circulation. In particular, when the body is at rest, the blood in the extremities returns to the liver. As an extension of this, it is said in Chinese medicine that the liver is yin in form but yang in function. Thus the liver requires sufficient blood to keep it *and its associated tissues* moist and supple, cool and relaxed.

3. The emotion associated with the liver is anger.

Anger is the emotion that typically arises when the liver is diseased and especially when its qi does not flow freely. Conversely, anger damages the liver. Thus the emotions related to the stagnation of qi in the liver are frustration, anger, and rage.

The spleen

The spleen is less important in Western medicine than it is in Chinese medicine. Since at least the Yuan dynasty (1280-1368 CE), the spleen has been one of the two most important viscera of Chinese medicine (the other being the kidneys). In Chinese medicine, the spleen plays a pivotal role in the creation of qi and blood and in the circulation and transformation of body fluids. Therefore, when it comes to the spleen, it is especially important not to think of this Chinese viscus in the same way as the Western spleen. The main statements of fact concerning the spleen and IBS in Chinese medicine are:

1. The spleen governs movement and transformation.

This refers to the movement and transformation of foods and liquids through the digestive system. In this case, movement and transformation may be paraphrased as digestion. This means that the spleen is the single most important viscus in Chinese medicine in all digestive processes and diseases. However, secondarily, movement and transformation also refer to the movement and transformation of body fluids through the body. It is the spleen qi which is largely responsible for controlling liquid metabolism in the body. If the spleen fails to move and transport body fluids properly, these may gather and accumulate and transform into "evil" or pathological dampness. Once engendered, this pathological dampness may further damage and weaken the spleen.

2. The spleen governs the muscles and flesh.

This statement is closely allied to the previous one. It is the constructive qi which constructs or nourishes the muscles and flesh. If there is sufficient spleen qi producing sufficient constructive qi, then the person's body is well fleshed and rounded. In addition, their muscles are normally strong. Conversely, if the spleen becomes weak, this may lead to emaciation and/or lack of strength.

3. The spleen governs the four limbs.

This means that the strength and function of the four limbs is closely associated with the spleen. If the spleen is healthy and strong, then there is sufficient strength in the four limbs and warmth in the four extremities. If the spleen becomes weak and insufficient, then there may be lack of strength in the four limbs, lack of warmth in the extremities, or even tingling and numbness in the extremities.

4. Thought is the emotion associated with the spleen.

In the West, we do not usually think of thought as an emotion per se. Be that as it may, in Chinese medicine, it is classified along with anger, joy, fear, fright, grief, and melancholy. In particular, thinking, or perhaps I should say overthinking, causes the spleen qi to bind. This means that the spleen qi does not flow harmoniously and this typically manifests as loss of appetite, abdominal bloating after meals, and indigestion.

5. The spleen is the source of engenderment and transformation.

Engenderment and transformation refer to the creation or production of the qi and blood out of the food and drink we take in each day. If the spleen receives adequate food and drink and then properly transforms that food and drink, it engenders or creates the qi and blood. The kidneys and lungs also participate in the creation of the qi, and the kidneys and heart participate in the creation of the blood, but the spleen is the pivotal viscus in both processes. Therefore, spleen qi weakness and insufficiency is a leading cause of qi and blood insufficiency and weakness.

6. The spleen governs upbearing of the clear.

The clear is the pure part of the digestate which the spleen sends up to the lungs to become the qi. If the clear is upborne, the turbid or impure part of the digestate is downborne.

7. The spleen is averse to dampness.

This means that either externally invading dampness or internally engendered dampness may damage the spleen and weaken its functions. Many foods, such as sugars and dairy products, engender fluids and, therefore, can cause or aggravate dampness which may then damage and weaken the spleen.

The stomach

1. The stomach governs the intake and decomposition of grain and water.

The stomach receives food and drink and begins the process of "ripening" or decomposing it, so that it can then be transformed by the spleen. The relatively impure or turbid portion of the digestate is borne downward by the stomach qi to the small intestine.

2. The stomach governs downbearing.

Just as the spleen qi governs upbearing, the stomach governs downbearing. This means that it is the stomach qi descending and downward movement which downbears the turbid part of the digestate to the intestines for excretion.

The large intestine

1. The large intestine governs the transformation and conveyance of waste.

In Chinese medicine, the large intestine controls the final reabsorption of nutrients and liquids from the digestate and then conveys the dregs of that process out of the body via defecation. Hence the large intestine completes the digestive process which the stomach begins by taking in food and liquids. Thus it is easy to see that disease processes in the large intestine may be begun in and influenced by whatever is going on in the viscera and bowels discussed above and which reside above it.

Above I mentioned that there are five viscera and six bowels. The sixth bowel is called the triple burner. It is said in Chinese that, "The triple burner has a function but no form." The name triple burner refers to the three main areas of the torso. The upper burner is the chest. The middle burner is the space from the bottom of the rib cage to the level of the navel. The lower burner is the lower abdomen below the navel. These three spaces are called burners because all of the functions and transformations of the viscera and bowels which they contain are "warm" transformations similar to food cooking in a pot on a stove or similar to an alchemical transformation in a furnace. In fact, the triple burner is nothing other than a generalized concept of how the other viscera and bowels function together as an organic unit in terms of the digestion of foods and liquids and the circulation and transformation of body fluids.

The Channels & Network Vessels

Each viscus and bowel has a corresponding channel with which it is connected. In Chinese medicine, the inside of the body is made up of the viscera and bowels. The outside of the body is composed of the sinews and bones, muscles and flesh, and skin and hair. It is the channels and network vessels (*i.e.*, smaller connecting vessels) which connect the inside and the outside of the body. It is through these channels and network vessels that the viscera and bowels connect with their corresponding body tissues.

The channels and network vessel system is a unique feature of traditional Chinese medicine. These channels and vessels are different from the circulatory, nervous, or lymphatic systems. The earliest reference to these channels and vessels is in *Nei Jing (Inner Classic)*, a text written around the second or third century BCE.

The channels and vessels perform two basic functions. They are the pathways by which the qi and blood circulate through the body and between the organs and tissues. Additionally, as mentioned above, the channels connect the viscera and bowels internally with the exterior part of the body. This channel and vessel system functions in the body much like the world information communication network. The channels allow the various parts of our body to cooperate and interact to maintain our lives.

This channel and network vessel system is complex. There are 12 primary channels, six yin and six yang, each with a specific pathway through the external body and connected with an internal organ (see diagram below). There are also extraordinary vessels, sinew channels, channel divergences, main network vessels, and ultimately countless finer and finer network vessels permeating the entire body. All of these form a closed loop or circuit similar to but distinct from the Western circulatory system.

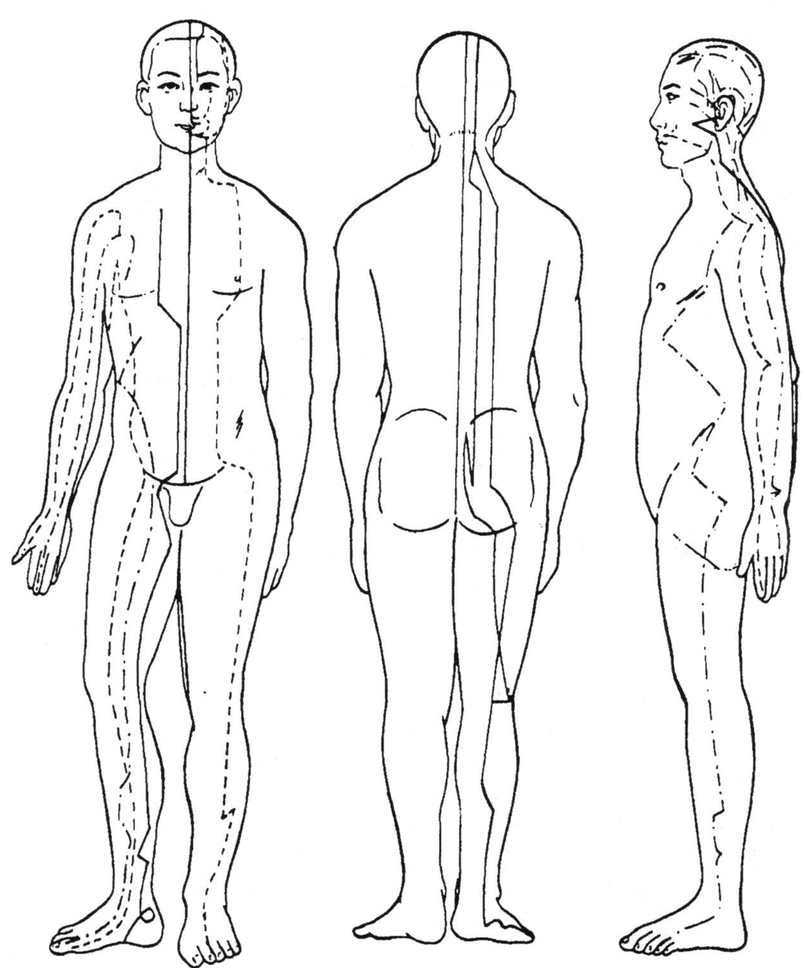

Acupuncture points are places located on the major channels where there is a special concentration of qi and blood. Because of the relatively more qi and blood accumulated at these places, the sites act as switches which can potentially control the flow of qi and blood in the channel on which the point is located. By stimulating these points in any of a number of different ways, one can speed up or slow down, make more or reduce, warm or cool down the qi and blood flowing in the channels and vessels. The main ways of stimulating these points and thus adjusting the flow of qi and blood in the channels and vessels is to needle them and to heat them by moxibustion.[1] Other commonly used ways of stimulating these points and thus adjusting the qi and blood flowing through the channels and vessels are massage, cupping, the application of magnets, and the application of various herbal medicinals. If the channels and vessels are the pathways over which the qi and blood flow, then the acupuncture points are the places where this flow can be adjusted.

[1] Moxibustion refers to adding heat to an acupuncture point or area of the body by burning a dried herb, Folium Artemisiae Argyii (*Ai Ye*), Oriental mugwort, on, over, or near the area to be warmed.

3
The Chinese Disease Mechanisms of IBS

Although Chinese doctors have been treating functional gastrointestinal complaints for centuries if not millennia, the term IBS is a relatively recent addition to the Chinese medical literature. In Chinese, irritable bowel syndrome is frequently translated as *guo min xing jie chang yan. Guo min xing* translated literally is "excessively responding type." This is the Chinese term for allergic. *Jie chang* literally means the knotted intestine and is the Chinese name for the colon. *Yan* means inflammation. Thus, this term may be translated as irritable colon or allergic colitis. Other names used for irritable bowel syndrome translate to urgent colon syndrome, mucous colitis, and spastic colitis. These are a modern Chinese attempt to literally translate IBS into Chinese. However, in older medical literature and according to traditional Chinese medical thought, the main symptoms of IBS are covered by the Chinese disease categories of constipation, diarrhea, and abdominal pain.

As I mentioned in the introduction and as anyone who suffers with IBS knows, the symptoms of the syndrome can include far more than the three listed above. Below is a list of some of the symptoms, both gastrointestinal and otherwise, that may be seen in people with IBS.

Abdominal pain
Abdominal bloating or distention
Constipation
Diarrhea
Alternating constipation and diarrhea
Flatulence
Nausea
Vomiting

A feeling that the bowel movement is incomplete
Mucous in the stools
Anal or rectal pain
Burning in or around the anus
Pelvic pain
Poor appetite
Headache
Fatigue
Lassitude
Anxiety
Depression
Irritability
Poor mental concentration
Backache
Bowel incontinence
Food intolerance and allergies
Belching
Heartburn
Feeling of a lump in the throat or trouble swallowing

Most people with IBS will have several of these complaints. In addition to the above symptoms, most of which are fairly common, any given patient with IBS may present with complaints that are idiosyncratic or unique to them. Even though a given symptom may not be recognized in Western medicine as part of the syndrome of IBS, in Chinese medicine *all* signs and symptoms are taken into account when developing a diagnosis and treatment plan. Thus Chinese medicine addresses all signs and symptoms associated with any person's IBS.

Disease causes, disease mechanisms

As we have seen, in Chinese medical theory, it is the stomach's job to receive food and drink and begin the digestive process by "rottening and ripening" it. Then it is the spleen's job to separate the pure from the impure and bear the pure part of the food and drink upward to the lungs where it becomes the qi and to the heart where it becomes the blood. The stomach then takes what is left (the impure or turbid portion) and transports it downward to the small intestine. Therefore, when the spleen and stomach are functioning properly the spleen qi tends to move upward and the stomach qi tends to move downward in a balanced and coordinated relationship with each other. This upward and downward flowing of the spleen and stomach qi is referred to as the qi mechanism. If the spleen does not correctly or adequately move untransformed food downward, resulting in symptoms such as lower abdominal distention or diarrhea. If stomach function is impaired, there is abnormal flow of qi upward and the turbid portion of the food is not transported downward, resulting in epigastric distention, nausea, belching, or constipation.

There are two reasons why the qi mechanism might not be working properly. The first has to do with the liver. As we have seen above, the liver controls coursing and discharge which means the free and smooth flow of qi to every part of the body. In Chinese medicine, the liver is called the "temperamental viscus." This means that it is easily damaged or upset by emotional influences. In particular, it is said that, "The liver likes orderly reaching." This means that the liver qi likes to spread out without restriction or hindrance like a large broad-leafed tree. When the liver encounters frustration, its coursing and discharging of the qi is inhibited. The qi cannot flow as freely as it wants and it becomes depressed and stagnant.

It is a fact of life that adults cannot do everything they want to do at the moment they want to do it. Delaying gratification is one of the things all adults learn, whether they like it or not. However, when we cannot do what we want to do when we want to do it, this affects our liver's coursing and discharging and the free spreading of our qi. It is a rare adult who has so few thwarted desires that their qi flows absolutely freely and uninhibitedly. Therefore, a certain level of liver depression qi stagnation is endemic in being an adult (at least in a civilized society where one must practice certain restraints) and, in actual clinical fact, almost all adults have some manifestations of liver depression qi stagnation.

When the qi becomes stagnant and bottled up, this gives rise to anger and irritability since anger is the emotion associated with Chinese liver disease. Since the liver governs the coursing and discharging of qi in the whole body, liver depression qi stagnation may also interfere with the normal upbearing and downbearing functions of the spleen and stomach qi, disrupting the qi mechanism and giving rise to the digestive symptoms mentioned above. When liver qi disrupts spleen function it is often referred to as "liver assailing the spleen," and, when it is stomach function that is affected, this is called "liver assailing the stomach."

The second reason that the qi mechanism might not be working properly has to do with the spleen. Overwork and improper diet, too much thinking or worrying, too much sitting, and not enough exercise all tend to weaken the spleen. Also, according to the *Nei Jing (Inner Classic)*, the "bible of Chinese medicine" compiled sometime in the second or third century BCE, the spleen and stomach begin to decline at around 35 years of age. Because the spleen and its helper, the stomach, are the source of the creation of qi and blood out of the food and liquids we eat, a decline in spleen-stomach function corresponds to a decline in the amounts of qi and blood produced. Qi provides the motivating force for all transportation and movement in the body. So when there is not enough qi, the spleen cannot transport the pure upward and the stomach cannot transport the turbid downward. Thus, a lack of qi may also lead to qi stagnation.

The modern Chinese medical literature is unanimous in saying that the root cause of IBS is always a disharmony between the liver and spleen. Due to emotional stress and frustration, the liver becomes depressed and the qi becomes stagnant. Due to worry, lack of exercise, overfatigue, or improper diet, the spleen becomes vacuous and weak. In Chinese medicine, it is said that the liver controls the spleen. This is because the functioning of the qi mechanism is dependent on the free flow of liver qi. Therefore if the liver becomes depressed, this can cause or worsen spleen vacuity or weakness. Conversely, if the spleen is vacuous and weak, this may allow the liver to become depressed, or it may worsen existing liver depression. This is because spleen qi vacuity may lead to qi stagnation as we have seen above, and also because the liver is dependent upon a sufficient supply of blood to nourish it so that it can perform its duty of controlling the coursing and discharge of the qi.

It is easy to see how closely these two viscera are related in terms of the free flow of the qi. The liver allows the qi to flow freely, but it is the spleen which is the ultimate source of the qi's power to move. Hence liver depression and spleen vacuity typically go hand in hand in clinical practice. In addition, because of their monthly loss of blood, women's spleens must work harder at producing blood than men's spleens must. This also predisposes women in particular towards a spleen insufficiency and explains why three times as many women as men suffer from IBS.

According to Chinese medical theory, if the liver becomes depressed and the qi stagnant, this may eventually transform into pathological heat. Remember that the qi is inherently warm. If the qi becomes stuck and accumulates, backing up under pressure, all this depressed and stagnant yang qi will transform into what is called transformative or depressive heat. Over time, this pathological heat, being by nature yang, will consume and dry out the blood, body fluids and kidney yin. Since, in Chinese medicine, yin is supposed to control yang, if kidney yin becomes vacuous and weak, liver yang may become hyperactive. Since fire burns upward and the heart and lungs are located above the liver, this pathological heat may also accumulate in the heart and/or lungs, disturbing either or both heart and lung function.

As mentioned above, since the spleen is the root of the engenderment and transformation of blood, if the spleen becomes weak, the blood may also become vacuous. Since some essence from the kidneys is required in order to make new blood, it is said in Chinese medicine that blood and essence share a common source. What this means in terms of disease mechanisms is that enduring blood vacuity may lead to insufficiency of kidney essence. This may aggravate any tendency to kidney yin vacuity already caused by damage due to enduring heat.

Because the spleen is also in charge of moving and transforming liquids, if the spleen becomes weak, water dampness may accumulate. Dampness which is yin, being thick, heavy and turbid, tends to percolate downward and may further block the free flow of qi which is yang, thus aggravating liver depression. Dampness may also give rise to depressive heat which then may cause the dampness to become damp heat. It is also possible for liver depression/transformative heat to stew the juices and give rise to damp heat.

In addition, if qi becomes stagnant and the spleen becomes weak, food stagnation is easily engendered. Food stagnation means food which sits in the stomach undigested. Such food stagnation may also transform into depressive heat.

If dampness due to the spleen not moving and transporting fluids gathers and endures, it may congeal into phlegm. However, phlegm may also be due to intense heat steaming and fuming the fluids, congealing them into phlegm like cooking pudding on a stove top. In either case, phlegm, being a yin depression, obstructs the free and uninhibited flow of qi and blood. It may lodge between the skin and flesh, in the channels and network vessels, and in what are known as the clear orifices of the heart and head. Phlegm blocking the clear orifices of the heart gives rise to mental emotional problems. The clear orifices of the head refer to the sensory organs of the eyes, ears, nose, and mouth. If phlegm blocks any of these, then there will be some disturbance in the function of the associated sense. For instance, if the orifices of the eyes are blocked by phlegm, then there will be vision problems. If the orifices of the ears are blocked, there will be hearing problems, etc.

If qi stagnation fails to move the blood, the blood will stop and become static. Thus, if liver depression is bad enough or lasts long enough, it may give rise to blood stasis. Static blood is like silt in the blood vessels, and like silt in a river or canal, it may eventually clog and obstruct the flow of blood in the affected area.

Blood stasis is mainly associated with pain, such as abdominal pain, headache, or other relatively severe aches and pains which are fixed in location and tend to be sharp or piercing in nature.

In Chinese medicine, the functioning of the spleen and stomach are likened to a pot on a stove and the process of digestion and the production of qi and blood is likened to the cooking of sour mash and distillation of alcohol. According to this metaphor, qi and blood are the distillation of foods and liquids cooked and transformed by the spleen and stomach. However, the ultimate source of heat for the spleen and stomach to do their job is the kidney fire or kidney yang. This kidney fire can be likened to the pilot light in a stove. If it goes out, the burners cannot function. Therefore, if the spleen remains chronically weak, since kidney yang is the source of the heat of the middle burner, *i.e.,* the spleen and stomach, kidney yang may also become weak. Since kidney essence is the material basis of both kidney yin and yang, this process can be accelerated if there is long-term blood vacuity. On the other hand, enduring kidney yang vacuity and weakness will also impair blood production as well.

All this may seem pretty complicated to the novice in Chinese medicine. As I said at the beginning of this book, Chinese medicine is a very complex system of thought. Even if one cannot grasp the meanings and implications of all of the above on their first reading, the reader should by now agree that Chinese medicine is by no means a primitive folk medicine. As we will see below, there are even a few more mechanisms which may occur as ramifications of these two disease mechanisms. However, liver depression qi stagnation and spleen qi vacuity are the mechanisms that are at the root of most irritable bowel signs and symptoms. If one understands these mechanisms and has a sound grasp of the basic theories of Chinese medicine discussed above, one can figure out *a rational explanation for any sign or symptom anyone may experience as a result of irritable bowel syndrome.*

4
Treatment According to Pattern Discrimination

The hallmark of professional Chinese medicine is what is known as "treatment based on pattern discrimination." Modern Western medicine bases its treatment on a disease diagnosis. This means that two patients diagnosed as suffering from the same disease will get the same treatment. Traditional Chinese medicine also takes the patient's disease diagnosis into account. However, the choice of treatment is not based on the disease so much as it is on what is called the patient's pattern, and it is treatment based on pattern discrimination which is what makes Chinese medicine the holistic, safe, and effective medicine it is.

In order to explain the difference between a disease and pattern, let us take headache for example. Everyone who is diagnosed as suffering from a headache has to, by definition, have some pain in their head. In modern Western medicine and other medical systems which primarily prescribe on the basis of a disease diagnosis, one can talk about "headache medicines." However, amongst headache sufferers, one may be a man and the other a woman. One may be old and the other young. One may be fat and the other skinny. One may have pain on the right side of her head and the other may have pain on the left. In one case, the pain may be throbbing and continuous, while the other person's pain may be very sharp but intermittent. In one case, they may also have indigestion, a tendency to loose stools, lack of warmth in their feet, red eyes, a dry mouth and desire for cold drinks, while the other person has a wet, weeping, crusty skin rash with red borders, a tendency to hay fever, ringing in their ears, and dizziness when they stand up. In Chinese medicine just as in modern Western medicine, both these patients suffer from headache. That is their disease diagnosis. However, they also suffer from a whole host of other complaints, have very different types of headaches, and very different constitutions, ages, and sex. In Chinese medicine, the patient's pattern is made up from all these other signs and symptoms and other information. Thus, in Chinese medicine, the pattern describes *the totality of the person as a unique individual.* And in Chinese medicine, treatment is designed to rebalance that entire pattern of imbalance as well as address the major complaint or disease. Thus, there is a saying in Chinese medicine:

> One disease, different treatments
> Different diseases, same treatment

This means that, in Chinese medicine, two patients with the same named disease diagnosis may receive different treatments *if their Chinese medical patterns are different*, while two patients diagnosed with different named diseases may receive the same treatment *if their Chinese medical pattern is the same.* In other words, in Chinese medicine, treatment is predicated primarily on one's pattern discrimination, not on one's named disease diagnosis. Therefore, each person is treated individually. There is no IBS formula or IBS herb. Nor is there any magic IBS acupuncture point.

Since every patient gets just the treatment which is right to restore balance to their particular body, there are also no unwanted side effects. Side effects come from forcing one part of the body to behave while causing an imbalance in some other part. The medicine may have fit part of the problem but not the entirety of the patient as an individual. This is like robbing Peter to pay Paul. Since Chinese medicine sees the entire body (and mind!) as a single, unified whole, curing imbalance in one area of the body while causing it in another is unacceptable.

Below is a description of the main Chinese medical patterns seen in patients with IBS:

Spleen qi vacuity

Main symptoms: Loose stools or diarrhea, increased frequency of bowel movements, especially after eating, reduced appetite, epigastric and abdominal distention and fullness, fatigue, loss of strength in the extremities, a pale facial complexion, a fat tongue with thin, white fur, and a fine, weak pulse

Treatment principles: Fortify the spleen and supplement the qi

Liver depression qi stagnation

Main symptoms: Constipation with small round stools which are not dry or diarrhea alternating with constipation, the urge to have a bowel movement but difficultly doing so, belching, chest, rib-side and/or abdominal distention or pain, mental depression, irritability, premenstrual breast distention and pain, a normal or slightly dark tongue with thin, white fur, and a bowstring[1] pulse

Treatment principles: Course the liver and rectify the qi

Although Chinese medical teachers like to present each pattern as a single, discreet entity, In actual clinical fact, these two patterns never present in this simple, discreet manner in IBS. According to my clinical experience and according to the Chinese medical literature, there is *always* some combination of both patterns. Therefore, in clinical practice, one chooses a prescription which remedies spleen vacuity if that is more pronounced and then modifies that for liver depression, while, if liver depression is the dominant pattern, then one chooses a formula for liver depression and modifies that for spleen vacuity. Or one

---

[1] There are 28 main pulse types in Chinese medicine, the bowstring pulse being one of these. It feels like its name implies—like a taut violin or bowstring.

chooses what is called a "harmonizing" formula which treats liver depression and spleen vacuity simultaneously.

The following patterns are seen in IBS as complications of the main two patterns presented above:

Spleen vacuity with dampness encumbrance

Main symptoms: All the signs and symptoms of spleen qi vacuity plus mucous in the stool, obesity, bodily heaviness, chest oppression, epigastric fullness, a fat, swollen tongue with teeth marks on its edges, white, possibly slimy tongue fur, and a slippery or fine, floating pulse

Treatment principles: Fortify the spleen and boost the qi plus penetrate turbidity and transform dampness

Spleen dampness is a complication of spleen qi vacuity. It is most often not listed as a separate pattern since most people with spleen qi vacuity have some degree of damp accumulation. However, in determining treatment, it is important to identify the degree of dampness present and modify the formula or acupuncture treatment accordingly.

Spleen vacuity with food stagnation

Main symptoms: The signs and symptoms of spleen qi vacuity plus more pronounced abdominal distention and a full feeling in the abdomen after eating, no thought for food or drink, loose, possibly putrid-smelling stools with undigested food, bad breath, slimy tongue fur, and a slippery pulse

Treatment principles: Fortify the spleen and supplement the qi, disperse food and abduct stagnation.

Depressive heat

Main symptoms: All the signs and symptoms of liver depression qi stagnation plus increased irritability, heart vexation (meaning an irritable, hot sensation in the upper abdomen and/or chest), a bitter taste in the mouth or acid eructations, a red tongue, especially on the sides, possibly swollen edges of the tongue, yellow fur, and a rapid, bowstring pulse

Treatment principles: Course the liver and rectify the qi, clear depressive heat

Damp heat

Main symptoms: Loose stools or diarrhea, possibly dark, green-colored stools, or light, yellow, mustard-colored stools, a burning or acid feeling around the anus with or after defecation, foul-smelling stools, slimy, yellow tongue fur, and a slippery, rapid pulse

Treatment principles: Clear heat and eliminate dampness

Kidney yang vacuity

Main symptoms: Possible daybreak diarrhea (*i.e.*, diarrhea very early in the morning), weakness or soreness in the low back or knees, decreased libido, frequent urination, waking at night to urinate, cold lower half of the body and especially the feet, a pale tongue with a thin, white coating, a deep, slow and forceless pulse

Treatment principles: Supplement the kidneys and invigorate yang

This pattern is a typical complication of IBS in older people. In women, it often shows up after 40 years of age. Since it complicates already existing liver depression qi stagnation and spleen qi vacuity it will not be seen clinically in the textbook form described above. Typically, as few as two or three of the symptoms of kidney yang vacuity will be present along with the symptoms of the main patterns. In particular, the tongue and pulse will tend to reflect the main patterns. Therefore, the tongue or at least its tip may actually be red and the pulse may be floating and fast as opposed to the standard textbook description of slow and deep.

Blood vacuity (of the large intestine, liver and/or heart)

Main symptoms: Constipation with dry stools, poor sleep, dry skin or hair, muscular stiffness, tension, or cramps, numbness in the extremities, blurred vision, night blindness, dizziness, heart palpitations, anxiety, poor memory, pale lips, a pale tongue with a slightly dry fur, and a fine pulse

Treatment principles: Nourish and supplement the blood

The signs and symptoms of blood vacuity vary depending on which viscera are affected. Pain, numbness, and vision problems are related to the liver. Constipation is obviously due to blood vacuity leading to fluid dryness in the large intestine. While heart blood vacuity is characterized by palpitations, poor memory, anxiety and disturbed sleep. The remainder of the symptoms are characteristic of blood vacuity in general.

Kidney yin vacuity/vacuity heat

Main symptoms: Low back pain and knee soreness, frequent but scanty, darkish urination, dizziness, tinnitus, early morning insomnia, night sweats, hot flashes, heat in the palms and soles of the feet, a red tongue with no or scanty fur, and a fine, rapid, or floating, rapid pulse

Treatment principles: Supplement the kidneys, enrich yin, and clear vacuity heat

The real deal

Although textbook discriminations such as the ones above make it seem like all the practitioner has to do is match up their patient's symptoms with one of the aforementioned patterns and then prescribe the recommended guiding formula, in actual clinical practice, one usually encounters combinations of the above discreet patterns and their related disease mechanisms or progressions. The main Chinese patterns the Chinese medical literature describes in terms of IBS and the ones I have encountered in my own patients are:

Liver depression qi stagnation
Depressive heat
Spleen qi vacuity
Spleen vacuity with damp encumbrance
Blood vacuity
Kidney yin vacuity with vacuity heat
Spleen-kidney yang vacuity
Large intestine fluid dryness
Replete heat in the heart, lungs, and/or stomach
Vacuity heat in the heart, lungs, and/or stomach
Heart qi and/or blood vacuity
Food stagnation
Blood stasis
Stomach & intestine damp heat

Given these patterns as the most common ones in IBS, it is also possible that some IBS patients might also have ascendant liver yang hyperactivity, liver fire flaring upward, internal stirring of liver wind, gallbladder timidity (*i.e.*, a combination of liver depression, spleen vacuity, and phlegm), heart-gallbladder dual vacuity (the same set of patterns as the preceding plus heart qi and/or heart blood vacuity), or phlegm fire. All these are evolutions or complications of liver depression.

As stated above, in all cases of IBS, spleen qi vacuity and liver depression qi stagnation play a central role. However, because of the interrelationships between the liver, the spleen, and all the other viscera and bowels of Chinese medicine and between the qi, blood, fluids, and essence, spleen weakness and liver depression may be complicated by or evolve into a number of other patterns. But, no matter what the combinations of patterns or their permutations, all a Chinese medical practitioner ever has to do is identify all these patterns, state the treatment principles for each pattern presented, and choose and administer treatments designed to achieve each of those therapeutic goals. Typically, when there is more than a single pattern, one first identifies the main disease mechanism currently at work and chooses a guiding formula or treatment based on rebalancing that imbalance. Then this guiding formula is modified to address all of the patient's associated disease mechanisms and signs and symptoms. However, if a mechanism or symptom will disappear by merely rebalancing some more fundamental mechanism, such secondary or dependent mechanisms and symptoms need not be addressed specifically.

All signs and symptoms of IBS can be diagnosed and treated according to Chinese medicine based on various combinations of the above disease mechanisms and patterns. In order to make this work, one must have a firm grasp of the defining or main symptoms of each pattern. Such a grasp is normally beyond most laypersons. Therefore, to get the full benefits of Chinese medicine, it is best if one receives a pattern discrimination from a qualified professional practitioner. Below I will discuss how and where to find such practitioners in the United States.

However, there is a lot one can do on one's own if one has only a general idea of their Chinese medical pattern. Hopefully, readers with IBS have identified some of their own signs and symptoms in the patterns discussed above. If so, see which pattern includes the majority of your signs and symptoms. Then write that down. It is probable that is the main pattern or disease mechanism accounting for your IBS. Even if you only address the main pattern and miss some of the minor complications, you should experience some relief of your symptoms. And remember, everyone with IBS has liver depression qi stagnation and spleen qi vacuity as their main Chinese patterns and disease mechanisms. So following the dietary, exercise, and lifestyle recommendations for those two patterns are universally helpful for sufferers of IBS.

5
How This System Works in Real Life

Using all the above information on the theory of Chinese medicine, the characteristics of the patterns, and their mechanisms, the practitioner of Chinese medicine is able to diagnose and, therefore, treat any complaint or combination of complaints that might occur in IBS.

Rosemary's case

Take Rosemary, for instance, whom I introduced at the beginning of this book. Rosemary is in her early 40s and has had symptoms of IBS off and on for many years. Rosemary's symptoms are always worse during periods of stress. On a bad day, she may have lower abdominal cramps and diarrhea 3-5 times per day. The cramping usually goes away after she goes to the bathroom. For Rosemary, episodes of diarrhea and cramps are triggered by eating. When her IBS is at its worst, they are particularly bad after she eats almost any raw fruits or vegetables, and she typically has diarrhea immediately after eating sweets. Sometimes there is mucous in the stools. Rosemary often feels bloated after she eats, occasionally she gets nauseous after she eats, and she doesn't have much of an appetite. Even so, she gains weight easily. Occasionally, Rosemary gets a headache on one side of her head which she attributes to tension and stress. These headaches make her extremely irritable. Rosemary is fatigued and feels as if she could sleep any time. Sometimes she has trouble working because she is light-headed and absentminded. Rosemary's tongue is pale and has a slimy, white coating. Her tongue is a little swollen, and one can see the indentations of her teeth along its edges. On light pressure, her pulse is bowstring, but on deeper pressure it feels slippery.

How a Chinese doctor analyzes Rosemary's symptoms

In Chinese medicine the spleen is responsible for transforming food and liquids and transporting the pure portion upward. Therefore, weakness of the spleen is one of the leading causes of diarrhea. In particular, diarrhea that is triggered by eating suggests spleen qi vacuity weakness. So the Chinese doctor immediately suspects that this is playing a part in Rosemary's IBS. This suspicion is confirmed by other signs and symptoms, such as Rosemary's fatigue. The spleen is the root of qi and blood production, and fatigue is *always* a symptom of qi vacuity or weakness. The fact that the spleen qi is weak and insufficient is also corroborated by the fact that Rosemary gets bloated after she eats. It is the spleen's job to "disperse and transform" the digestate, and, if it is weak, it cannot do this. Thus there is indigestion. In addition, Rosemary is intolerant to raw and sweet foods. In Chinese medicine, uncooked foods are considered particularly difficult to digest. Therefore, eating raw foods tends to aggravate any condition due to a weak spleen. Sweet is the flavor which "gathers" in the spleen, and sweet is a "supplementing" flavor, engendering both more qi and more fluids. A little sweet flavor supplements the spleen qi, but too much actually damages the spleen further and leads to the formation of internal dampness.

In addition to weakness of the spleen, Rosemary's IBS also involves liver depression qi stagnation. We have seen that the liver is easily damaged by emotional influences which impair the free flow of the qi. Rosemary's condition always worsens when she is experiencing mental-emotional stress. Another sign of liver depression is abdominal pain. In Chinese medicine, it is a given that:

If there is pain, there is no free flow.
If there is free flow, there is no pain.

Since there is cramping, we know that the flow of qi is not free and easy. The bowel movement is itself a type of discharge. Therefore, after bowel movements, the qi is free to flow again and the pain disappears. Headaches are another symptom which may be due to liver depression. When the qi becomes depressed and stagnant, it may accumulate and then counterflow upward. Headaches on one side of the head are characteristic of this abnormal upward counterflow of liver qi. In Rosemary's case, the headaches are accompanied by irritability. In Chinese, irritability is called "easy anger" and in Chinese medicine anger is the emotion of the liver. This is further evidence that the headaches are due to liver depression. Finally, a bowstring pulse is "the pulse of the liver" and is the definitive pulse image denoting liver depression and constraint.

As we already know, the spleen is responsible for moving and transforming body fluids. If the spleen qi is weak, these body fluids accumulate and transform into dampness, and if spleen vacuity persists for a long time, this dampness may eventually congeal into phlegm. Mucous in the stool is a sign of dampness and phlegm as is obesity. Adipose tissue in Chinese medicine is considered an accumulation of phlegm and dampness. Rosemary's pulse and tongue also indicate dampness and phlegm. A slippery pulse may denote the presence of heat or of other accumulations such as food stagnation, but, in Rosemary's case, given the other signs and symptoms, it confirms the presence of phlegm dampness. In addition, Rosemary's tongue is swollen with the indentations of her teeth along the edges and the tongue coating is slimy. Both the swollen, edematous tongue and a slimy coating are considered to be the result of the accumulation of dampness and phlegm.

When liver depression qi stagnation causes the qi to counterflow upward, it may draft this phlegm and dampness with it to the head. Rosemary's feelings of sleepiness, light-headedness, and absentmindedness or poor memory are, in part, caused by this combination of phlegm dampness and liver qi. Nausea is also a symptom caused by the upward counterflow of qi, in this case stomach qi. This may also be due to liver depression resulting in the liver's assailing the stomach with the stomach qi's losing its descending and downbearing. Again, phlegm and dampness being drafted upward with the qi may contribute to the nausea.

Therefore, based on the above signs and symptoms, the Chinese doctor knows that Rosemary's IBS is a combination of several factors: 1) spleen qi vacuity , 2) liver depression qi stagnation, and 3) accumulation of dampness and phlegm.

How a Chinese doctor treats Rosemary's IBS

Once a Chinese doctor knows the patient's pattern discrimination, the next step is to formulate the treatment principles necessary to rebalance the imbalance implied by this pattern discrimination. If the Chinese doctor listed spleen qi vacuity as number one in their pattern discrimination, then the first treatment principles are to fortify the spleen and boost the qi. These are the treatment principles for correcting a spleen qi vacuity. Fortifying the spleen means to strengthen its functions of transforming and moving. To boost the qi means to supplement or add to it and also to promote the upbearing of the clear or pure part of the digestate. If the second element in the pattern discrimination is liver depression qi stagnation, then the Chinese doctor knows that the second set of principles are to course the liver and rectify the qi. To course the liver means to promote the liver's coursing and discharge or spreading of the qi freely and easily throughout the body. Rectifying the qi means to make the qi move and, more than that, make it move in the right directions. Finally, if the third element in the pattern discrimination is the accumulation of dampness and phlegm, then the necessary treatment principles for rebalancing that are transforming phlegm and eliminating dampness.

Once the Chinese doctor has stated their treatment principles, then they know that anything which works to accomplish these principles will be good for the patient. Using these principles, the Chinese doctor can now select various acupuncture points which achieve these effects. They can prescribe Chinese herbal medicinals which embody these principles. They can make recommendations about what to eat and not eat based on these principles. They can make recommendations on lifestyle changes. And, in short, they can advise the patient on any and every aspect of their life, judging whether something either aids the accomplishment of these principles or works against it.

In Chinese medicine, the internal administration of Chinese (herbal)[1] medicinals is the main modality. So let's look at how a Chinese doctor crafts a prescription for Rosemary. Because the spleen is weak and the liver is depressed, the Chinese doctor knows there is a disharmony between the liver and spleen and, therefore, knows to pick the starting formula from the "harmonizing" category of Chinese medicinal formulas.[2] Further, the harmonizing formula must be one which courses the liver, rectifies the qi, fortifies the spleen, supplements the qi and eliminates dampness. (Some other harmonizing formulas harmonize the spleen and stomach, the stomach and intestines, or the inside of the body with the outside.)

Of the various formulas found in the harmonization chapter of the Chinese doctor's book of formulas and prescriptions, there is only one famous one which does just these things and treats abdominal cramping and diarrhea. It is called *Tong Xie Yao Fang*

---

1 I've put the word herbal in parentheses since Chinese medicine is not entirely herbal. Herbs are medicinals made from parts of plants, their roots, bark, stems, leaves, flowers, etc. Chinese medicinals are mostly herbal in nature. However, a percentage of Chinese medicinals also come from the animal and mineral realms. Thus not all Chinese medicinals are, strictly speaking, herbs.

2 In Chinese medicine, depending on the textbook, there are anywhere from 22-28 different categories of formulas.

(Painful Diarrhea Essential Formula). Let's look at its ingredients. This formula is composed of:

stir-fried Rhizoma Atractylodis Macrocephalae (*Bai Zhu*)[3]
stir-fried Radix Albus Paeoniae Lactiflorae (*Bai Shao*)
stir-fried Pericarpium Citri Reticulatae (*Chen Pi*)
Radix Ledebouriellae Divaricatae (*Fang Feng*)

Rhizoma Atractylodis Macrocephalae or White Atractylodes fortifies the spleen, supplements the qi, and dries dampness.[4] When it is stir-fried, it also stops diarrhea. Radix Albus Paeoniae Lactiflorae or White Peony soothes the liver and harmonizes the spleen, stops pain and stops diarrhea. Together, these two medicinals supplement the spleen and control the liver. Pericarpium Citri Reticulatae or Aged Orange Peel assists Atractylodes in drying dampness. In addition, it transforms phlegm and harmonizes the center. Radix Ledebouriellae Divaricatae or Ledebouriella courses the liver and rectifies the qi, moves the qi and dispels intestinal wind (*i.e.*, rumbling in the intestines).

Hence one can see that the ingredients in this formula very precisely and specifically embody and carry out the treatment principles we have said are necessary for rebalancing Rosemary's

---

[3] Stir-frying a medicinal means to heat it in a wok until it turns yellow or scorched. Stir-frying these medicinals enhances their effects of fortifying the spleen, transforming dampness, and relieving cramping.

[4] Because most Chinese medicinals have no commonly recognized English names, I identify these medicinals at least the first time they are introduced first by their Latin pharmacological identification followed by their Chinese name in parentheses. If the "herb" in question has a well-known common English name, the next time I refer to that ingredient, I first use the Latin followed by the common name. In subsequent instances, I then just use the common English name.

condition. In actual fact, this formula is very often used as the starting formula when treating IBS *as long as it presents as liver depression and spleen vacuity.* This formula is not an "IBS formula" *per se.* Its choice has less to do with the disease diagnosis and everything to do with the Chinese pattern discrimination. If the Chinese doctor viewed Rosemary's condition as a result of spleen qi vacuity and felt that the liver depression was merely a complicating factor, he might have chosen a formula from the qi-supplementing category and then modified it to treat liver qi. Thus, the goal in choosing a Chinese herbal formula is not so much to treat this disease or that. Rather, it is to treat people with a particular set of patterns who happen to also have certain diagnosed diseases.

To make this formula even more effective, the Chinese doctor will also rarely prescribe it in the textbook form above. Rather, he will modify it by taking out one or more ingredients and adding others as necessary in order to tailor it to the individual patient's exact configuration of signs and symptoms. Since Rosemary's case is due primarily to spleen qi vacuity and she is particularly fatigued, I would add Radix Panacis Ginseng (*Ren Shen*) and Radix Astragali Membranacei (*Huang Qi*). These are the most famous spleen-fortifying qi supplements in Chinese medicine. Dampness is also a large part of Rosemary's case. So I might also add a medicinal such as Semen Coicis Lachryma-jobi (*Yi Yi Ren*) to stop diarrhea by fortifying the spleen and seeping dampness. To increase the effect of coursing the liver and rectifying the qi and, therefore, more effectively stop cramping and pain, I would add Radix Aucklandiae Lappae (*Mu Xiang*). This medicinal promotes the movement of qi in the intestines, stops lower abdominal pain, and assists the other medicinals in stopping diarrhea and strengthen the transforming and moving functions of the spleen. Another ingredient I would add to treat phlegm dampness would be Rhizoma Pinelliae Ternatae (*Ban Xia*). Rhizoma Pinelliae Ternatae or Pinellia dries dampness, transforms phlegm, and harmonizes the middle burner, meaning the spleen and stomach. It is particularly useful in treating nausea. Finally, mix-fried Radix Glycyrrhizae (*Gan Cao*) or Licorice may be added to help Ginseng and Pinellia fortify the spleen and supplement the qi. In addition, Licorice moderates any harsh actions of any of the other medicinals in the formula and helps these other medicinals to act in a concerted and harmonious way.

Whenever possible, we try to use the least number of ingredients which do the most of what is required. Usually, I would start with something as close to the basic formula as possible and then modify it as needed during the course of treatment. However, there is no limit to the modifications I might make to this formula in order to make it match perfectly Rosemary's exact signs and symptoms, constitution, and tolerances.

The ingredients in this formula may be dispensed in bulk and then brewed as a "tea" by the patient or may be taken as a dried, powdered extract. Many standard formulas also come as ready-made pills. However, these cannot be modified. If their ingredients match the individual patient's requirements, then they are fine. If the formula needs modifications, then teas or powders whose individual ingredients can be added and subtracted are necessary.

In exactly the same way, the Chinese doctor could create an individualized acupuncture treatment plan and would certainly create an accompanying dietary and lifestyle plan. However, we will discuss each of these in their own chapter. In a woman Rosemary's age with her Chinese pattern discrimination, Chinese herbal medicine alone or combined with acupuncture and supported by the proper diet and lifestyle will usually eliminate or at the very least drastically diminish her IBS within three months of treatment.

6
Chinese Herbal Medicine and IBS

As we have seen from Rosemary's case above, there is no Chinese "IBS herb" or even "IBS formula." Chinese medicinals are individually prescribed based on a person's pattern discrimination, not on a disease diagnosis like IBS. The pattern discrimination is very important because if, for example, a person has IBS and almost all of his symptoms are due to liver depression, then too many qi supplements or too high a dose of them will make the person feel worse, not better. Since this person's qi is depressed, adding more qi to what is already not flowing freely only adds to this depression and may worsen the symptoms that are due to it, such as abdominal pain, constipation, or irritability.

In addition, because most people with IBS present with more than one Chinese pattern and disease mechanism, professional Chinese medicine never treats those with IBS with herbal "singles." In Western herbalism, singles mean the prescription of a single herb all by itself. Chinese herbal medicine is based on rebalancing patterns, and patterns in real-life patients almost always have more than a single element. Therefore, Chinese doctors almost always prescribe herbs in multi-ingredient formulas. Such formulas may have anywhere from six to eighteen or more ingredients. When a Chinese doctor reads a prescription by another Chinese doctor, they can tell you not only what the patient's pattern discrimination is but also their probable signs and symptoms. In other words, the Chinese doctor does not just combine several medicinals which are all reputed to be "good for IBS." Rather, they carefully craft a formula whose ingredients are meant to rebalance every aspect of the patient's body–mind.

Getting your own individualized prescription

In China, it takes not less than four years of full-time college education to learn how to do a professional Chinese pattern discrimination and then write an herbal formula based on that pattern discrimination, most laypeople cannot realistically write their own Chinese herbal prescriptions. It should also be remembered that Chinese herbs are not effective and safe because they are either Chinese or herbal. In fact, approximately 20% of the common Chinese materia medica did not originate in China, and not all Chinese herbs are completely safe. They are only safe when prescribed according to a correct pattern discrimination, in the right dose, and for the right amount of time. After all, if an herb is strong enough to heal an imbalance, it is also strong enough to create an imbalance if overdosed or misprescribed. Therefore, I strongly recommend that those who wish to experience the many benefits of Chinese herbal medicine see a qualified professional practitioner who can do a professional pattern discrimination and write an individualized prescription. Towards the end of this book, I will give suggestions on how to find such a practitioner.

Experimenting with Chinese patent medicines

In reality, qualified professional practitioners of Chinese medicine are not yet found in every North American community. In addition, some people may want to try to heal their IBS as much on their own as possible. More and more health food stores are stocking a variety of ready-made Chinese formulas in pill and powder form. These ready-made, over-the-counter Chinese medicines are often referred to as Chinese patent medicines. Although my best recommendation is for people to seek Chinese herbal treatment from professional practitioners, below are some suggestions of how one might experiment with Chinese patent medicines to treat IBS.

In Chapter 4, I have given the signs and symptoms of the two key or basic patterns associated with most cases of IBS. These are:

1. Spleen qi vacuity
2. Liver depression qi stagnation

And I have discussed seven common complicating patterns:

1. Spleen vacuity with damp encumbrance
2. Spleen vacuity with food stagnation
3. Depressive heat
4. Kidney yang vacuity
5. Blood vacuity
6. Kidney yin vacuity with vacuity heat
7. Damp heat

The first step in choosing a formula is to identify the main pattern or patterns causing your IBS. After you have done that, you can consider trying one or more of the following Chinese patent remedies.

Tong Xie Yao Fang

As mentioned above, *Tong Xie Yao Fang* means "Painful Diarrhea Essential Formula." Happily, this famous formula for spleen vacuity and liver depression with abdominal cramping and diarrhea is now available in pill form as well as a desiccated extract powder. This is the single most commonly prescribed Chinese medicinal formula for IBS. We have already described its ingredients and discussed their functions in the preceding chapter. If a person only presented with a very simple pattern of spleen vacuity and liver depression, one could try this formula all by itself. However, that is rarely the case. Also happily, this formula can be combined with other ready-made, Chinese patent medicines which then treat other simultaneously presenting patterns.

If, for any reason, this formula or any of those discussed below causes any side effects, please stop its use and seek the counsel of a qualified professional practitioner of Chinese medicine. Chinese medicine is supposed to heal without any side effects. Side effects are an indication that a medicine is not totally right for you.

Xiao Yao Wan

Xiao Yao Wan is used for abdominal pain and chronic constipation from liver depression qi stagnation, particularly in women. Its Chinese name has been translated as "Free & Easy Pills," "Rambling Pills," "Relaxed Wanderer Pills," and several other versions of this same idea of promoting a freer and smoother, more relaxed flow. As a patent medicine, this formula comes as both pills and desiccated powdered extract.

The ingredients in this formula are:

Radix Bupleuri (*Chai Hu*)
Radix Angelicae Sinensis (*Dang Gui*)
Radix Albus Paeoniae Lactiflorae (*Bai Shao*)
Rhizoma Atractylodis Macrocephalae (*Bai Zhu*)
Sclerotium Poriae Cocos (*Fu Ling*)
mix-fried Radix Glycyrrhizae (*Gan Cao*)
Herba Menthae Haplocalycis (*Bo He*)
uncooked Rhizoma Zingiberis (*Sheng Jiang*)

This formula treats the pattern of liver depression qi stagnation complicated by blood vacuity and spleen vacuity with possible dampness as well. Radix Bupleuri or Bupleurum courses the liver and rectifies the qi. It is aided in this by Herba Menthae Haplocalycis or Peppermint. Radix Angelicae Sinensis or Dang Gui and White Peony nourish the blood and soften and harmonize the liver. Atractylodes and Sclerotium Poriae Cocos or Poria fortify the spleen and eliminate dampness. Mix-fried Licorice aids these two in fortifying the spleen and supplementing the liver, while Rhizoma Zingiberis or uncooked Ginger aids in both promoting and regulating the qi flow and eliminating dampness.

When IBS presents with the signs and symptoms of liver depression and spleen vacuity with blood vacuity and more dampness, one can try taking this formula along with *Tong Xie Yao Fang Wan* described above.

Dan Zhi Xiao Yao Wan

Dan Zhi Xiao Yao Wan or "Moutan & Gardenia Rambling Pills" is a modification of the above formula which also comes as a patent medicine in the form of pills and also as a desiccated powdered extract. It is meant to treat the pattern of liver depression transforming into heat with spleen vacuity and possible blood vacuity and/or dampness. The ingredients in this formula are the same as above except that two other herbs are added:

Cortex Radicis Moutan (*Dan Pi*)
Fructus Gardeniae Jasminoidis (*Shan Zhi Zi*)

These two ingredients clear heat and resolve depression. In addition, Cortex Radicis Moutan or Moutan quickens the blood and dispels stasis and is good at clearing heat specifically from the blood. Some Chinese doctors say to take out uncooked Ginger and Mint from the *Xiao Yao Wan*, while others leave these two ingredients in.

Basically, the signs and symptoms of the pattern for which this formula is designed are the same as those for *Xiao Yao Wan* above plus signs and symptoms of depressive heat. These might include a reddish tongue with slightly yellow fur, a bowstring and rapid pulse, a bitter taste in the mouth, and increased irritability.

When depressive heat complicates a liver-spleen disharmony, one can try combining these pills with *Tong Xie Yao Fang Wan* described above.

Mu Xiang Shun Qi Wan

Mu Xiang Shun Qi Wan is used for constipation, abdominal fullness and abdominal pain. It comes in both pill and powdered extract forms. Its name means "Auklandia Normalize the Qi Pills." It is appropriate to use when liver depression qi stagnation is more pronounced and is complicated by food stagnation as well. Unlike *Xiao Yao Wan* above, it does not nourish the blood and it supplements the spleen only slightly. Its ingredients are:

Radix Aucklandiae Lappae (*Mu Xiang*)
Semen Alpiniae Katsumadai (*Dou Kou*)
Rhizoma Atractylodis (*Cang Zhu*)
uncooked Rhizoma Zingiberis Officinalis (*Sheng Jiang*)
Pericarpium Citri Reticulatae Viride (*Qing Pi*)
Pericarpium Citri Reticulatae (*Chen Pi*)
Sclerotium Poriae Cocos (*Fu Ling*)
Radix Bupleuri (*Chai Hu*)
Cortex Magnoliae Officinalis (*Hou Po*)
Semen Arecae Catechu (*Bing Lang*)
Fructus Citri Aurantii (*Zhi Ke*)
Radix Linderae Strychnifoliae (*Wu Yao*)
Semen Raphani Sativi (*Lai Fu Zi*)
Fructus Crataegi (*Shan Zha*)
Massa Medica Fermentatae (*Shen Qu*)
Fructus Germinatus Hordei Vulgaris (*Mai Ya*)
Radix Glycyrrhizae (*Gan Cao*)

Most of the ingredients in this formula rectify and move the liver qi. However, Semen Raphani or Radish Seeds, Fructus Crataegi or Hawthorn Fruit, Massa Medica Fermentata or Medicated Leaven, and Fructus Germinatus Hordei Vulgaris or Malted Barley all disperse food accumulation. White Atractylodes and Poria fortify the spleen and disinhibit dampness.

One can try combining this formula with *Tong Xie Yao Fang Wan* when liver depression qi stagnation is the main pattern and abdominal cramping and distention are the main symptoms. If taking these pills causes feelings of dryness or heat internally or if they make one even more vexed and irritable, either their dosage should be reduced or they should be stopped. Women who are nursing should not take this formula because it contains Malted Barley, a very effective medicinal for stopping lactation.

Shu Gan Wan

Shu Gan Wan means "Soothe the Liver Pills." I believe it is only available in pill form at the present time. This Chinese patent medicine is made up almost entirely of liver-coursing and qi-rectifying medicinals. However, instead of also including food stagnation medicinals, it includes several medicinals which dry and transform dampness. Its ingredients are:

Fructus Meliae Toosendan (*Chuan Lian Zi*)
Rhizoma Curcumae Longae (*Jiang Huang*)
Lignum Aquilariae Agallochae (*Chen Xiang*)
Rhizoma Corydalis Yanhusuo (*Yan Hu Suo*)
Radix Aucklandiae Lappae (*Mu Xiang*)
Semen Alpiniae Katsumadai (*Dou Kou*)
Radix Albus Paeoniae Lactiflorae (*Bai Shao*)
Sclerotium Poriae Cocos (*Fu Ling*)
Fructus Citri Aurantii (*Zhi Ke*)
Pericarpium Citri Reticulatae (*Chen Pi*)
Fructus Amomi (*Sha Ren*)
Cortex Magnoliae Officinalis (*Hou Po*)

This formula can be combined with *Tong Xie Yao Fang Wan* when IBS consists of liver depression with more dampness. The symptoms of this might include abdominal distention and cramping and more nausea and even vomiting or burping and belching. As with the previous formula, these pills should be discontinued if there are feelings of dryness, heat or increased irritability.

Shen Ling Bai Zhu Wan

Shen Ling Bai Zhu Wan means "Ginseng, Poria & Atractylodes Pills." This is the guiding formula for treating diarrhea due to spleen qi vacuity with dampness. It comes as a Chinese-made patent medicine in pill form and is also available as a powdered extract. Its ingredients are:

Radix Codonopsitis Pilosulae (*Dang Shen*)
Rhizoma Atractylodis Macrocephalae (*Bai Zhu*)
Sclerotium Poriae Cocos (*Fu Ling*)
mix-fried Radix Glycyrrhizae (*Gan Cao)*
Radix Dioscoreae Oppositae (*Shan Yao*)
Semen Dolichoris Lablab (*Bai Bian Dou*)
Semen Nelumbinis Nuciferae (*Lian Zi*)
Semen Coicis Lachryma-jobi (*Yi Yi Ren*)
Fructus Amomi (*Sha Ren*)
Radix Platycodi Grandiflorae (*Jie Geng*)

This formula fortifies the spleen, supplements the qi, disinhibits dampness and stops diarrhea. Radix Codonopsitis Pilosulae or Codonopsis and Radix Dioscoreae Oppositae or Dioscorea supplement the qi. White Atractylodes, Poria, and Semen Coicis Lachryma-jobi or Coix fortify the spleen and seep dampness. Semen Dolichoris Lablab or Dolichos and Semen Nelumbinis Nuciferae or Lotus Seed fortify the spleen and stop diarrhea.

Shen Ling Bai Zhu Wan is an extremely effective formula for stopping diarrhea when it is caused by spleen qi vacuity and dampness. However, it is rare to see an individual with irritable bowel syndrome who does not have at least a little liver depression qi stagnation even if the spleen is very weak. For this reason, it is usually necessary to combine this formula with some other formula. For instance, by combining it with *Tong Xie Yao Fang Wan*, it now treats liver-spleen disharmony as well.

By combining this formula with *Mu Xiang Shun Qi Wan* one can treat spleen qi vacuity, spleen dampness, liver depression qi stagnation, and food stagnation. If there is more spleen qi vacuity use relatively more *Shen Ling Bai Zhu Wan*. If there is more liver qi use a greater amount of *Mu Xiang Shun Qi Wan*. One could also add a small amount of *Xiao Yao Wan* to *Shen Ling Bai Zhu Wan* if the main pattern is spleen qi vacuity with dampness with a little bit of liver depression and blood vacuity.

The presence of a significant degree of dampness due to spleen vacuity is the key criteria for choosing *Shen Ling Bai Zhu Wan*. It is not appropriate if there are pronounced signs of dryness or heat, and it should be used with caution or modified if blood vacuity is a large part of the pattern.

Xiang Sha Liu Jun Zi Wan

The name of these pills translates as "Auklandia & Amomum Six Gentlemen Pills." This formula is currently available in the West as both ready-made pills and powdered extract. It treats the pattern of pronounced spleen vacuity with elements of dampness and a little qi stagnation. These pills can be taken along with *Xiao Yao Wan* in those cases where spleen vacuity is more severe. These pills are especially good for treating poor appetite, nausea, abdominal bloating after meals, and loose stools due to spleen vacuity and dampness. Their ingredients include:

Radix Codonopsitis Pilosulae (*Dang Shen*)
Rhizoma Atractylodis Macrocephalae (*Bai Zhu*)
Sclerotium Poriae Cocos (*Fu Ling*)
Rhizoma Pinelliae Ternatae (*Ban Xia*)

mix-fried Radix Glycyrrhizae (*Gan Cao*)
Pericarpium Citri Reticulatae (*Chen Pi*)
Radix Auklandiae Lappae (*Mu Xiang*)
Fructus Amomi (*Sha Ren*)

One should not take these pills, however, if there are signs of damp heat such as burning around the anus with bowel movements or diarrhea with dark colored, foul-smelling, explosive stools.

Ren Shen Jian Pi Wan

The ingredients in these pills include:

Radix Codonopsitis Pilosulae (*Dang Shen*)
Fructus Crataegi (*Shan Zha*)
Rhizoma Atractylodis Macrocephalae (*Bai Zhu*)
Fructus Immaturus Citri Aurantii (*Zhi Shi*)
Pericarpium Citri Reticulatae (*Chen Pi*)
Fructus Germinatus Hordei Vulgaris (*Mai Ya*)

The name of this formula means "Ginseng Fortify the Spleen Pills," and it treats spleen qi vacuity with food stagnation. It can be used combined with *Tong Xie Yao Fang Wan, Shen Ling Bai Zhu San, Xiao Yao Wan* and/or *Dan Zhi Xiao Yao Wan* in order to strengthen any one of those medicines' ability to supplement the spleen and disperse food stagnation. It also contains Malted Barley and so is contraindicated for nursing mothers. I believe this formula only comes in pill form at the present time.

Ren Shen Lu Rong Wan

These pills contain:

Radix Panacis Ginseng (*Ren Shen*)
Cortex Eucommiae Ulmoidis (*Du Zhong*)
Radix Morindae Officinalis (*Ba Ji Tian*)

Radix Astragali Membranacei (*Huang Qi*)
Cornu Parnum Cervi (*Lu Rong*)
Radix Angelicae Sinensis (*Dang Gui*)
Radix Achyranthis Bidentatae (*Niu Xi*)
Arillus Euphoriae Longanae (*Long Yan Rou*)

Ren Shen Lu Rong Wan means "Ginseng & Deer Antler Pills." This formula treats spleen-kidney yang vacuity, and, in IBS, kidney yang vacuity is only seen complicating a spleen qi vacuity. This combined pattern is a progression of spleen qi vacuity and is usually seen in those in their middle to late 40s or older. Therefore, this formula can be combined with *Tong Xie Yao Fang Wan* when spleen-kidney yang vacuity complicates liver-spleen disharmony. This formula is only currently available in pill form in the West.

Run Chang Wan

Semen Cannabis Sativae (*Huo Ma Ren*)
Semen Pruni Persicae (*Tao Ren*)
Herba Cistanchis Deserticolae (*Rou Cong Rong*)
Radix Angelicae Sinensis (*Dang Gui*)
Radix Et Rhizoma Rhei (*Da Huang*)

Run Chang Wan means "Moisten the Intestines Pills." These pills clear heat and nourish the blood, moisten the intestines and free the flow of the stools. They are used to treat large intestine fluid dryness constipation.[1] This formula may be added to those used for the main pattern if the stools are hard and dry. Because this patent medicine contains Radix Et Rhizoma Rhei or Rhubarb, which is a strong purgative, it should not be used for long periods of time. It should also not be taken if one has diarrhea or loose

[1] When sold as a dried, powdered extract, this formula is called Linum and Rhubarb Combination.

stools. If it causes diarrhea, its use should be discontinued immediately.

Bu Zhong Yi Qi Wan

Bu Zhong Yi Qi Wan means "Supplement the Center & Boost the Qi Pills." This formula is available from a wide variety of suppliers in both pill and powdered extract form. It treats the pattern of central qi vacuity or central qi downward fall. The central qi is another name for the spleen and stomach qi. This formula is especially good for treating spleen vacuity weakness manifesting not so much as digestive complaints and diarrhea but as more pronounced fatigue and orthostatic hypotension. Orthostatic hypotension means dizziness on standing up. The ingredients in this formula are:

Radix Astragali Membranacei (*Huang Qi*)
Radix Codonopsitis Pilosulae (*Dang Shen*)
Rhizoma Atractylodis Macrocephalae (*Bai Zhu*)
mix-fried Radix Glycyrrhizae (*Gan Cao*)
Radix Angelicae Sinensis (*Dang Gui*)
Radix Bupleuri (*Chai Hu*)
Rhizoma Cimicifugae (*Sheng Ma*)
Pericarpium Citri Reticulatae (*Chen Pi*)
Fructus Zizyphi Jujubae (*Da Zao*)
uncooked Rhizoma Zingiberis (*Sheng Jiang*)

This is actually a very sophisticated formula and it has a very wide range of application. It can be added to other formulas when spleen vacuity causing fatigue is more pronounced.

Ba Zhen Wan

Ba Zhen Wan literally means "Eight Pearls Pills." However, these are also often marketed under the name Women's Precious Pills. They are called "eight pearls" because they include four ingredients which supplement the qi and four ingredients which nourish the blood. These pills can be combined with *Tong Xie Yao Fang Wan* when there is liver depression complicated by more serious spleen qi and liver blood vacuity. They also might be added, for example, if the stools are dry even though there may be pronounced spleen qi vacuity. This formula is available in both powdered extract and pill form. The ingredients in this formula are:

Radix Codonopsitis Pilosulae (*Dang Shen*)
Rhizoma Atractylodis Macrocephalae (*Bai Zhu*)
Sclerotium Poriae Cocos (*Fu Ling*)
mix-fried Radix Glycyrrhizae (*Gan Cao*)
Radix Angelicae Sinensis (*Dang Gui*)
Radix Albus Paeoniae Lactiflorae (*Bai Shao*)
cooked Radix Rehmanniae (*Shu Di*)
Radix Ligustici Wallichii (*Chuan Xiong*)

Do *not* take this formula if there is marked diarrhea.

Suan Zao Ren Tang

Suan Zao Ren Tang means "Zizyphus Seed Decoction." It is available in both pill and powdered extract form. It treats insomnia and mental unrest due to liver blood vacuity. It can, therefore, be combined with *Tong Xie Yao Fang Wan* when heart-liver blood vacuity is more severe and manifests primarily as insomnia. Its ingredients are:

Semen Zizyphi Spinosae (*Suan Zao Ren*)
Sclerotium Poriae Cocos (*Fu Ling*)
Radix Ligustici Wallichii (*Chuan Xiong*)
Rhizoma Anemarrhenae Aspheloidis (*Zhi Mu*)
mix-fried Radix Glycyrrhizae (*Gan Cao*)

Gui Pi Wan

Gui means to return or restore, *pi* means the spleen, and *wan* means pills. Therefore, the name of these pills means "Restore the Spleen Pills." This formula is available in both pill and powdered extract form. However, these pills not only supplement the spleen qi but also nourish heart blood and calm the heart spirit. They are the textbook guiding formula for the pattern of heart-spleen dual vacuity. In this case, there are symptoms of spleen qi vacuity, such as fatigue, poor appetite, and cold hands and feet, plus symptoms of heart blood vacuity, such as a pale tongue, heart palpitations, anxiety, emotional withdrawal, and insomnia. This formula is also the standard one for treating heavy or abnormal bleeding due to the spleen not containing and restraining the blood within its vessels. This patent medicine would not be used as the main formula in treating IBS but could be added to *Tong Xie Yao Fang Wan*, for example, to treat mental-emotional symptoms caused by liver depression qi stagnation and spleen qi vacuity complicated with heart blood vacuity. Its ingredients are:

Radix Astragali Membranacei (*Huang Qi*)
Radix Codonopsitis Pilosulae (*Dang Shen*)
Rhizoma Atractylodis Macrocephalae (*Bai Zhu*)
Sclerotium Pararadicis Poriae Cocos (*Fu Shen*)
mix-fried Radix Glycyrrhizae (*Gan Cao*)
Radix Angelicae Sinensis (*Dang Gui*)
Semen Zizyphi Spinosae (*Suan Zao Ren*)
Arillus Euphoriae Longanae (*Long Yan Rou*)
Radix Polygalae Tenuifoliae (*Yuan Zhi*)
Radix Auklandiae Lappae (*Mu Xiang*)

Er Chen Wan

Er Chen Wan means "Two Aged (Ingredients) Pills." This is because two of its main ingredients are aged before using. This formula is used to transform phlegm and eliminate dampness. It can be added to *Tong Xie Yao Fang Wan* if there is liver depression with spleen vacuity and more pronounced phlegm and dampness. This formula is available from a wide variety of suppliers in both pill and powdered extract form. Its ingredients include:

Rhizoma Pinelliae Ternatae (*Ban Xia*)
Sclerotium Poriae Cocos (*Fu Ling*)
mix-fried Radix Glycyrrhizae (*Gan Cao*)
Pericarpium Citri Reticulatae (*Chen Pi*)
uncooked Rhizoma Zingiberis (*Sheng Jiang*)

Bai Tou Weng Tang

Bai Tou Weng is the Chinese name of the main ingredient in this formula, Radix Pulsatillae Chinensis. *Tang* means "decoction." This formula is available in desiccated powdered extract form. It is the main Chinese medicinal formula for large intestine damp heat diarrhea. Its ingredients *in toto* are:

Radix Pulsatillae Chinensis (*Bai Tou Weng*)
Rhizoma Coptidis Chinensis (*Huang Lian*)
Cortex Fraxini (*Qin Pi*)
Cortex Phellodendri (*Huang Bai*)

This medicine can be added to *Tong Xie Yao Fang Wan* or other Chinese ready-made medicines when IBS is complicated by damp heat.

Ban Xia Xie Xin Wan

Ban Xia Xie Xin Wan means "Pinellia Drain the Heart Pills." This formula harmonizes the spleen and stomach and stomach and intestines when there is both spleen vacuity and damp heat. It now comes as both pills and powdered extract. It is comprised of:

Rhizoma Pinelliae Ternatae (*Ban Xia*)
Radix Codonopsitis Pilosulae (*Dang Shen*)
dry Rhizoma Zingiberis (*Gan Jiang*)
mix-fried Radix Glycyrrhizae (*Gan Cao*)
Rhizoma Coptidis Chinensis (*Huang Lian*)
Radix Scutellariae Baicalensis (*Huang Qin*)

It can be combined with *Tong Xie Yao Fang Wan* when liver-spleen disharmony is complicated by damp heat, but not as much damp heat as the preceding medicine treats.

Xiao Chai Hu Tang Wan

The name of this medicine means "Minor Bupleurum Decoction Pills." It is a liver-spleen, spleen-stomach harmonizing medicine. It can be combined with *Tong Xie Yao Fang Wan* when there is even less damp heat or when there is only heat in the stomach and/or lungs. This formula is available in both pill and powdered extract form. Its ingredients are:

Radix Bupleuri (*Chai Hu*)
Radix Codonopsitis Pilosulae (*Dang Shen*)
Rhizoma Pinelliae Ternatae (*Ban Xia*)
Radix Scutellariae Baicalensis (*Huang Qin*)
mix-fried Radix Glycyrrhizae (*Gan Cao*)
uncooked Rhizoma Zingiberis (*Sheng Jiang*)
Fructus Zizyphi Jujubae (*Da Zao*)

Yu Quan Wan

The name of this medicine translates as "Jade Spring Pills." As far as I know, it is only available in pill form. This medicine can be taken along with *Tong Xie Yao Fang* or some other formula when there is pronounced yin vacuity. Its ingredients are:

Radix Trichosanthis Kirlowii (*Tian Hua Fen*)
Tuber Ophiopogonis Japonici (*Mai Men Dong*)
Sclerotium Poriae Cocos (*Fu Ling*)

Radix Astragali Membranacei (*Huang Qi*)
Radix Codonopsitis Pilosulae (*Dang Shen*)
cooked Radix Rehmanniae (*Shu Di*)
Fructus Pruni Mume (*Wu Mei*)
Fructus Schisandrae Chinensis (*Wu Wei Zi*)
Radix Puerariae (*Ge Gen*)
Radix Glycyrrhizae (*Gan Cao*)

Sometimes, yin-supplementing medicinals can cause or aggravate diarrhea. Unfortunately, spleen qi vacuity and yin vacuity often go together if damp or depressive heat has consumed and damaged yin fluids or due to age. I have chosen this formula for combination with *Tong Xie Yao Fang* or other of the above formulas because it contains several anti-diarrhea Chinese medicinals. Therefore, it is less likely to cause loose stools or aggravate diarrhea than any other yin-supplementing and enriching Chinese ready-made I know.

Where to order the above Chinese medicines

The pill forms of the above Chinese patent medicines can be ordered directly from either of two companies:

Mayway Corp.
1338 Mandela Parkway
Oakland, CA 94607 USA
Tel: 1-800-2- MAYWAY
Fax: 1-800-909-2828
email: sales@mayway.com
Website: www.mayway.com

Nuherbs Co.
3820 Penniman Ave.
Oakland, CA 94619 USA
Tel: 510-534-4372 / 800-233-4307
Fax: 510-534-4384 / 800-550-1928

Desiccated powdered extracts of many of the above Chinese medicinal formulas are available from:

Qualiherb/Finemost Corp.
13340 E. Firestone Blvd. #N
Santa Fe Springs, CA 90670 USA
Tel: 1-800-533-5907

Side effects

The above Chinese patent medicines only give a suggestion of how one or several over-the-counter Chinese ready-made medicines may be used to treat IBS. As a professional practitioner of Chinese medicine, I prefer to see people receive a professional diagnosis and an individually tailored prescription. However, as long as one is careful to try to match up their pattern with the right formula and not to exceed the recommended dosage on each medicine's package, one can try treating their IBS with one or more of these remedies. If it works, great! These patent medicines are usually quite cheap compared to Western prescription drugs. If this approach doesn't work after three months or if there are *any side effects*, one should stop and see a professional practitioner.

In general, you can tell if any medication and treatment are good for you by checking the following six guideposts.

1. Digestion
2. Elimination
3. Energy level
4. Mood
5. Appetite
6. Sleep

If a medication, be it modern Western or traditional Chinese, gets rid of your symptoms and all six of these basic areas of human health improve or are fine to begin with, then that medicine or treatment is probably OK. However, even if a treatment or medication takes away your major complaint, if it causes deterioration in one of these six basic parameters, then that treatment or medication is probably not OK and is certainly not OK for long–term use. When medicines and treatments, even so-called natural, herbal medications, are prescribed based on a person's pattern of disharmony, then there is healing without side effects. According to Chinese medicine, this is the only kind of true healing.

7
Acupuncture & Moxibustion

When the average Westerner thinks of Chinese medicine, they probably first think of acupuncture. Certainly acupuncture is the best known of the various methods of treatment which go to make up Chinese medicine. However, in China, acupuncture is actually a secondary treatment modality, most Chinese immediately thinking of "herbal" medicine when thinking of Chinese medicine.

Be that as it may, most professional practitioners of Chinese medicine in North America are licensed or otherwise registered and permitted to practice medicine as acupuncturists. Therefore, most such practitioners treat every patient with at least some acupuncture no matter if they also prescribe a Chinese herbal formula as well. While this "doubling up" of these two therapies is not always necessary to successfully treat IBS, IBS in general does respond very well to correctly prescribed and administered acupuncture.

What is acupuncture?

Acupuncture primarily means the insertion of extremely thin, sterilized, stainless steel needles into specific points on the body where Chinese doctors have known for centuries there are special concentrations of qi and blood. Therefore, these points are like switches or circuit breakers for regulating and balancing the flow of qi and blood over the channel and network system we described above. As we have seen, IBS is always at least partially due to liver depression qi stagnation. This means that it is a disease due to the erroneous flow of qi. Because the qi is depressed and stagnant, it is not flowing when and where it should. Instead it counterflows or vents itself to areas of the body where it shouldn't be, attacking other organs and body tissues and making them dysfunctional.

Therefore, IBS typically includes signs and symptoms associated with lack of, or erroneous, counterflow qi flow. Since acupuncture's forte is the regulation and rectification of the flow of qi (and, thus secondarily, the blood), it is an especially good treatment mode for correcting diseases due to liver depression qi stagnation. In that case, insertion of acupuncture needles at various points in the body moves stagnant qi in the liver and leads the qi to flow in its proper directions and amounts.

As a generic term, acupuncture also includes several other methods of stimulating acupuncture points, thus regulating the flow of qi in the body. The main other modality is moxibustion. This means the warming of acupuncture points mainly by burning dried, aged Oriental mugwort on, near, or over acupuncture points. The purpose of this warming treatment are to 1) even more strongly stimulate the flow of qi and blood, 2) add warmth to areas of the body which are too cold, and 3) add yang qi to the body to supplement a yang qi deficiency. Other acupuncture modalities are to apply suction cups over points, to massage the points, to prick the points to allow a drop or two of blood to exit, to apply Chinese medicinals to the points, to apply magnets to the points, and to stimulate the points by either electricity or laser.

What is a typical acupuncture treatment for IBS like?

In China, acupuncture treatments are given every day or every other day. After a course of 10 treatments there is a break of a few days and then another course of 10 treatments is started. In the United States, some practitioners will treat two or three times in a week in the beginning of a case or if there are really acute symptoms, such as diarrhea, but most treat once a week.

When acupuncture is combined with Chinese herbal medicine, this more relaxed treatment schedule seems to work OK.

When a person comes for an appointment, the practitioner will ask what the main symptoms are, will typically look at the tongue and its fur, and will feel the pulses at the radial arteries on both wrists. Then, they will ask the patient to lie down on a treatment table. Based on their Chinese pattern discrimination, the practitioner will select anywhere from one to eight or nine points to be needled.

The needles used today are ethylene oxide gas sterilized disposable needles. This means that they are used one time and then thrown away, just like a hypodermic syringe in a doctor's office. However, unlike relatively fat hypodermic needles, acupuncture needles are hardly thicker than a strand of hair. The skin over the point is disinfected with alcohol and the needle is quickly and deftly inserted somewhere typically between one quarter and a half inch. In some few cases, a needle may be inserted deeper than that, but most needles are only inserted relatively shallowly.

After the needle has broken the skin, the acupuncturist will usually manipulate the needle in various ways until he or she feels that the qi has "arrived." This refers to a subtle but very real feeling of resistance around the needle. When the qi arrives, the patient will usually feel a mild, dull soreness around the needle, a slight electrical feeling, a heavy feeling, or a numb or tingly feeling. All these mean that the needle has tapped the qi and that treatment will be effective. Once the qi has been tapped, then the practitioner may further adjust the qi flow by manipulating the needle in certain ways, may attach the needle to an electro-acupuncture machine in order to stimulate the point with very mild and gentle electricity, or they may simply leave the needle in place. Usually the needles are left in place from 10-20 minutes. After this, the needles are withdrawn and thrown away. *Thus there is absolutely no chance for cross-infection from another patient.*

How are the points selected?

The points one's acupuncturist chooses to needle each treatment are selected on the basis of Chinese medical theory and the known clinical effects of certain points. Since there are different schools or styles of acupuncture, point selection tends to vary from practitioner to practitioner. However, let me present a fairly typical case from the point of view of the dominant style of acupuncture in the People's Republic of China.

Let's say the patient is a woman whose main complaints are alternating constipation and diarrhea. She has abdominal cramping after she eats, abdominal bloating, and fatigue. Her tongue is pale and slightly swollen and her pulse is fine and bowstring. Her Chinese pattern discrimination is constipation and abdominal pain due to liver depression qi stagnation and loose stools, abdominal bloating and fatigue due to spleen qi vacuity. This pattern is referred to as a disharmony of the liver and the spleen, which, as we have seen above, is typically the main pattern exhibited in people with IBS.

The treatment principles necessary for remedying this case are to course the liver and rectify the qi, fortify the spleen and supplement the qi. In addition, when the patient is having constipation, the practitioner will add the treatment principles of descending, precipitating, and freeing the flow of the stools. When the patient is having diarrhea, the treatment principle added is simply to stop diarrhea. In order to accomplish these aims, the practitioner might select the following points:

Tai Chong (Liver 3)
He Gu (Large Intestine 4)
Zu San Li (Stomach 36)
Tian Shu (Stomach 25)
Pi Shu (Bladder 20)
Wei Shu (Bladder 21)

When there is constipation, some selection or all of the following points might also be used:

Da Heng (Spleen 15)
Da Chang Shu (Large Intestine 25)
Zhi Gou (Triple Burner 6)
Yang Ling Quan (Gallbladder 34)

In that case, typically Bladder 20 and 21 are often omitted, since the presence of constipation as opposed to diarrhea usually suggests more liver depression and even some heat and less spleen vacuity. If there is significant concomitant constipation, of course, these points may be kept or they may be replaced with *Bai Hui* (Governing Vessel 20), thus substituting a single point for the two.

In the case of diarrhea, one or a selection of the following points might be added to the original prescription above:

Da Chang Shu (Bladder 25)
Shang Ju Xu (Stomach 37)
Nei Ting (Stomach 45)

Bladder 25 can be used for either constipation or diarrhea since it directly connects with the large intestine. If diarrhea is due to damp heat, one might choose St 37, while if there is dry heat in the stomach and intestines, St. 45 is a good choice.

In the original formula above, Liver 3 and Large Intestine 4 course the liver, rectify the qi, and disinhibit and harmonize the qi mechanism of the entire body. Therefore, this combination is called the "Four Gates." Large Intestine 4 and Stomach 36 strongly and effectively regulate and rectify the stomach and intestines. Stomach 36 also has an ability to supplement a vacuous, weak spleen and is especially indicated for fatigue. Stomach 25 directly connects to the large intestine and can normalize the flow of the large intestine qi, whether there is constipation or diarrhea or even if there is simply intestinal cramping. And the combination of Bladder 20 and 21 strongly supplements spleen vacuity.

In terms of the modifications of this basic formula for liver-spleen disharmony with intestinal irritability, Spleen 15 is located directly over the large intestine and is a good choice for more pronounced constipation. Large Intestine 25 connects directly with the large intestine and can treat both constipation and diarrhea. Triple Burner 6 and Gallbladder 34 rectify the qi of the liver via the gallbladder channel that is paired with the liver. They are also extremely empirically effective for qi stagnation constipation.

Thus these various combinations of six to a dozen points address this woman's Chinese pattern discrimination and her major complaints of constipation, diarrhea, pain, bloating and fatigue. They remedy both the underlying disease mechanism and address certain key symptoms in a very direct and immediate way. Hence they provide symptomatic relief *at the same time as* they correct the underlying mechanisms of these symptoms.

Does acupuncture hurt?

In Chinese, it is said that acupuncture is *bu tong*, painless. However, most patients will feel some mild soreness, heaviness, electrical tingling, or distention. When done well and sensitively, it should not be sharp, biting, burning, or really painful.

How quickly will I feel the result?

One of the best things about the acupuncture treatment of IBS is that its effects are immediate. Since some of the symptoms of IBS have to do with stuck qi, as soon as the qi is made to flow, the symptoms disappear. Therefore, for some IBS complaints, such as abdominal distention, headache, low back pain, lower abdominal cramps, or epigastric pain, *one will feel relief during the treatment itself.*

In addition, because feelings of being "stressed out" and nervous tension are also mostly due to liver depression qi stagnation, most people will feel an immediate relief of stress and tension while still on the table. Typically, one will feel a pronounced tranquility and relaxation within five to ten minutes of the insertion of the needles.

Who should get acupuncture?

As mentioned above, because most professional practitioners in the West are legally entitled to practice under various acupuncture laws, most acupuncturists will routinely do acupuncture on every patient. Since acupuncture's effects on IBS are usually so immediate, this is usually a good thing for IBS sufferers. However, acupuncture is particularly effective for abdominal distention and pain, and even if one is prescribed Chinese herbal medicinals for these complaints, one should consider a course of acupuncture in addition. Because acupuncture treats pain so effectively and immediately, one should consider receiving acupuncture especially for any IBS complaints associated with pain. And because acupuncture treats mental-emotional tension so well and so immediately, those with these types of symptoms should also get at least one course of acupuncture therapy.

When IBS symptoms mostly have to do with qi vacuity or blood vacuity, then acupuncture is not as effective as internally administered Chinese herbal medicinals. Although moxibustion can add yang qi to the body (and I will teach a home remedy for this in a separate section on moxibustion below), acupuncture needles cannot add qi, blood, or yin to a body in short supply of these. The best acupuncture can do in these cases is to stimulate the various viscera and bowels which engender and transform the qi, blood, and yin. Chinese herbs, on the other hand, can directly introduce qi and blood into the body, thus supplementing vacuities and insufficiencies of these. In IBS cases where qi and blood, vacuities are pronounced, one should either use acupuncture with Chinese medicinals or rely on Chinese medicinals alone. When there is pronounced yang vacuity complicating a liver-spleen disharmony, one can use moxibustion and needles with or without Chinese medicinals, but one should not use needles alone.

Ear acupuncture

Acupuncturists believe there is a map of the entire body in the ear and that by stimulating the corresponding points in the ear, one can remedy those areas and functions of the body. Therefore, many acupuncturists will not only needle points on the body at large but also select one or more points on the ear. In terms of IBS, needling the ear point *Shen Men* (Spirit Gate) can have a profound effect on relaxing tension and irritability and improving sleep. There are also ear points for the liver, spleen, stomach, and large intestine.

The nice thing about ear acupuncture points is that one can use tiny "press needles" which are shaped like miniature thumb tacks. These are pressed into the points, covered with adhesive tape, and left in place for five to seven days. This method can provide continuous treatment between regularly scheduled office visits. Thus ear acupuncture is a nice way of extending the duration of an acupuncture treatment. In addition, these ear points can also be stimulated with small metal pellets, radish seeds, or tiny magnets, thus getting the benefits of stimulating these points without having to insert actual needles.

8
The Three Free Therapies

Although one can experiment cautiously with Chinese herbal medicinals, one cannot really do acupuncture on oneself. Therefore, Chinese herbal medicine and acupuncture and its related modalities mostly require the aid of a professional practitioner. However, there are three free therapies which are crucial to preventing and treating IBS. These are diet, exercise, and deep relaxation.

Remember that the root causes of IBS are liver depression qi stagnation with concomitant spleen vacuity weakness. Liver depression is primarily due to stress and emotional factors, while spleen vacuity is primarily due to faulty diet. Of these three free therapies, therefore, diet is designed to cure the spleen, and exercise and relaxation are meant to cure the liver. When all three are coordinated, then they eliminate the causes and disease mechanisms of IBS. Since Western diets are, by Chinese medical standards, typically poor and since Western society tends to be both excessively sedentary and excessively stressful, lack of proper management of these three basic realms of human life is the reason why so many people in the West suffer from IBS. In other words, although IBS has been around for millennia, its incidence is probably higher now in the West because of relatively recent changes in our diet and lifestyle.

Diet

As discussed earlier, in Chinese medicine, the function of the spleen and stomach are likened to a pot on a stove or still. The stomach receives the foods and liquids which then "rotten and ripen" like a mash in a fermentation vat. The spleen then cooks this mash and drives off (*i.e.*, transforms and upbears) the pure part. This pure part collects in the lungs to become the qi and in the heart to become the blood. In addition, Chinese medicine characterizes this transformation as a process of yang qi transforming yin substance. All the principles of Chinese dietary therapy, including what people with IBS should and should not eat, are derived from these basic "facts."

We have seen that a healthy spleen is vitally important for keeping the liver in check and the qi freely flowing. We have also seen that the spleen is the root of qi and blood transformation and engenderment. Therefore, it is vitally important for those with IBS to avoid foods which damage the spleen and to eat foods which promote a healthy spleen and qi and blood production.

Foods which damage the spleen

In terms of foods which damage the spleen, Chinese medicine begins with uncooked, chilled foods. If the process of digestion is likened to cooking, then cooking is nothing other than predigestion outside of the body. In Chinese medicine, it is a given that the overwhelming majority of all food should be cooked, *i.e.*, predigested. Although cooking may destroy some vital nutrients (in Chinese, qi), cooking does render the remaining nutrients much more easily assimilable. Therefore, even though some nutrients have been lost, the net absorption of nutrients is greater with cooked foods than raw. Further, eating raw foods makes the spleen work harder and thus wears the spleen out more quickly. If one's spleen is very robust, eating uncooked, raw foods may not be so damaging, but we have already seen that in IBS the spleen is almost always already weak.

More importantly, chilled foods directly damage the spleen. Chilled, frozen foods and drinks neutralize the spleen's yang qi. The process of digestion is the process of warming all foods and drinks to 100° Fahrenheit within the stomach so that it may undergo transformation. If the spleen expends too much yang qi just warming the food up, then it will become damaged and weak. Therefore, all foods and liquids should be eaten and drunk at room temperature at the least and better at body temperature.

The more signs and symptoms of spleen vacuity a person presents, such as fatigue, chronically loose stools, undigested food in the stools, cold hands and feet, dizziness on standing up, and aversion to cold, the more important it is to avoid uncooked, chilled foods and drinks.

In addition, sugars and sweets directly damage the spleen. This is because sweet is the flavor which inherently "enters" the spleen. It is also an inherently dampening flavor according to Chinese medicine. This means that the body engenders or secretes fluids which gather and collect, transforming into dampness, in response to foods with an excessively sweet flavor. In Chinese medicine, it is said that the spleen is averse to dampness. Dampness is yin and controls or checks yang qi. The spleen's function is based on the transformative and transporting functions of yang qi. Therefore, anything which is excessively dampening can damage the spleen. The sweeter a food is, the more dampening and, therefore, more damaging it is to the spleen.

Another group of foods which are dampening and, therefore, damaging to the spleen is what Chinese doctors call "sodden wheat foods." This means flour products such as bread and noodles. Wheat (as opposed to rice) is damp by nature. When wheat is steamed, yeasted, and/or refined, it becomes even more dampening. In addition, all oils and fats are damp by nature and, hence, may damage the spleen. The more oily or greasy a food is, the worse it is for the spleen. Because milk contains a lot of fat, dairy products are another spleen-damaging, dampness-engendering food. This includes milk, butter, and cheese.

If we put this all together, then ice cream is just about the worst thing a person with a weak, damp spleen could eat. Ice cream is chilled, it is intensely sweet, and it is filled with fat. Therefore, it is a triple whammy when it comes to damaging the spleen. Likewise, pasta smothered in tomato sauce and cheese is a recipe for disaster. Pasta made from wheat flour is dampening, tomatoes are dampening, and cheese is dampening. In addition, what many people don't know is that a glass of fruit juice contains as much sugar as a candy bar, and, therefore, is also very damp-engendering and damaging to the spleen.

Below is a list of specific Western foods which damage the spleen because they are either uncooked, chilled, too sweet, or too dampening. In people with IBS consumption of these foods should be minimized or avoided in proportion to the degree of weakness and dampness of the spleen.

Ice cream
Sugar
Candy, especially chocolate
Milk
Butter
Cheese
Margarine
Yogurt
Raw salads
Fruit juices
Nuts
Juicy, sweet fruits, such as oranges, peaches, strawberries, and tomatoes
Fatty meats
Fried foods
Refined flour products
Yeasted bread
Alcohol (which is essentially sugar)

If the spleen is weak and wet, one should also not eat too much at any one time. A weak spleen can be overwhelmed by a large meal, especially if any of the food is hard-to-digest. This then results in food stagnation which only impedes the free flow of qi all the more and further damages the spleen.

A clear, bland diet

In Chinese medicine, the best diet for the spleen and, therefore, by extension for most humans, is what is called a "clear, bland diet." This is a diet high in complex carbohydrates such as unrefined grains, especially rice, and beans. It is a diet which is high in *lightly cooked* vegetables. It is a diet which is low in fatty meats, oily, greasy, fried foods, and very sweet foods. However, it is not a completely vegetarian diet. Most people, in my experience, should eat one to two ounces of various types of meat two to four times per week. This animal flesh may be the highly popular but overtouted chicken and fish, but should also include some lean beef, pork, and lamb. Some fresh or cooked fruits may be eaten, but fruit juices should be avoided. In addition, one should make an effort to include tofu and tempeh, two soy foods now commonly available in North American grocery food stores.

If the spleen is weak, then one should eat several smaller meals rather than one or two large meals. In addition, because rice is 1) neutral in temperature, 2) it fortifies the spleen and supplements the qi, and 3) it eliminates dampness, rice should be the main or staple grain in the diet.

A few problem foods

There are a few "problem" foods which deserve special mention. The first of these is coffee. Many people crave coffee for two reasons. First, coffee moves stuck qi. Therefore, in a person who suffers from liver depression qi stagnation, coffee will temporarily provide the feeling that the qi is flowing. Secondly, coffee transforms essence into qi and makes that qi temporarily available to the body. Therefore, those who suffer from spleen and/or kidney vacuity fatigue will get a temporary lift from coffee. They will feel like they have energy. However, once this energy is used up, they are left with a negative deficit. The coffee has transformed some of the essence stored in the kidneys into qi. This qi has been used, and now there is less stored essence. Since the blood and essence share a common source, coffee drinking may ultimately worsen any symptoms of IBS associated with blood or kidney vacuities.

Another problem food is chocolate. Chocolate is a combination of oil, sugar, and cocoa. We have seen that both oil and sugar are dampening and damaging to the spleen. Temporarily, the sugar will boost the spleen qi, but ultimately it will result in "sugar blues" or a hypoglycemic let-down. Cocoa stirs the life gate fire.

The life gate fire is another name for kidney yang or kidney fire, and kidney fire is the source of sexual energy and desire. It is said that chocolate is the food of love, and from the Chinese medical point of view, that is true. Since chocolate stimulates kidney fire at the same time as it temporarily boosts the spleen, it does give one rush of yang qi. In addition, this rush of yang qi does move depression and stagnation, at least short-term. So it makes sense that some people with liver depression, spleen vacuity, and kidney yang debility might crave chocolate.

Alcohol is both damp and hot according to Chinese medical theory. It strongly moves the qi and blood. Therefore, persons with liver depression qi stagnation will feel temporarily better from drinking alcohol. However, the sugar in alcohol damages the spleen and engenders dampness which "gums up the works," while the heat (yang) in alcohol can waste the blood (yin) and aggravate or inflame depressive liver heat.

Spicy, peppery, "hot" foods also move the qi, thereby giving some temporary relief to liver depression qi stagnation. However, like alcohol, the heat in spicy hot foods wastes the blood and can inflame yang.

In Chinese medicine, the sour flavor is inherently astringing and constricting. Therefore, people with IBS should limit their intake of vinegar and other intensely sour foods. Such sour-flavored foods may aggravate the qi stagnation by astringing and restricting the qi and blood all the more. This is also why sweet and sour foods, such as orange juice and tomatoes are particularly bad those with liver depression/spleen vacuity. The sour flavor astringes and constricts the qi, while the sweet flavor damages the spleen and engenders dampness.

Candidiasis & IBS

If one looks at the foods which I have recommended to minimize or avoid above and what I have recommended to eat, one will see that it comes very close or is identical to an anti-candida diet.

Polysystemic chronic candidiasis (PSCC) refers to a chronic overgrowth of yeasts and fungi in the body which then goes on to affect many different systems in the body. The pathological changes associated with PSCC are due to a combination of food allergies, immune system dysregulation, and autoimmune reactions. These pathological changes may affect the adrenals, pituitary gland, and thyroid gland, and in women, the ovaries. In the West, a tendency towards PSCC is due to faulty diet as outlined above, overuse of antibiotics, and overuse of hormone-based medicine from oral birth control pills to corticosteroids. From a Chinese medical point of view, this then results in deep-seated spleen vacuity with damp encumbrance usually complicated by liver depression and possibly by phlegm fluids, damp heat, and/or blood stasis in addition. Kidney yang vacuity may also develop if the spleen vacuity goes on for long enough or simply as a result of aging.

If a person with IBS has a history of multiple fungal and yeast infections, a history of recurrent or enduring antibiotic use (such as for recurrent bladder infections, acne or pelvic inflammatory disease), has a history of hormones used as medicine, or suffers from allergies, PSCC should be suspected as a component of that person's IBS. In that case, it is necessary to pay particular attention to the diet. The good news is that professionally prescribed Chinese herbal medicine can help remedy PSCC faster than just diet alone. The bad news is that, without proper diet, no amount of Chinese herbs will completely and permanently remedy this condition.

Some last words on diet

In conclusion, there are no magic foods that cure IBS. Diet most definitely plays a major role in the cause and perpetuation of IBS, but the issue is mainly what to avoid or minimize, not what to eat. Most of us know that coffee, chocolate, sugars and sweets, oils and fats, and alcohol are not good for us. Most of us know that we should be eating more complex carbohydrates and freshly cooked vegetables and less fatty meats. However, it's one thing to know these things and another to follow what we know.

To be perfectly honest, a clear bland diet *à la* Chinese medicine is not the most exciting diet in the world. It is the traditional diet of most lower and lower middle class peoples around the world living in temperate climates. It is the traditional diet of most of my readers' great grandparents. The point I am making here is that our modern Western diet which is high in oils and fats, high in sugars and sweets, high in animal proteins, and proportionally high in uncooked, chilled foods and drinks is a relatively recent aberration, and you can't fool Mother Nature.

When one switches to the clear, bland diet of Chinese medicine, at first one may suffer from cravings for more "flavorful" food. These cravings are, in many cases, actually associated with food "allergies." In other words, we may crave what is actually not good for us similar to an alcoholic craving alcohol. After a few days, these cravings tend to disappear and we may be amazed that we don't miss some of our convenience or "comfort" foods as much as we thought we would. If one has been addicted to a food like sugar for many years, it does not take much to "fall off the wagon" and be addicted again. Therefore, perseverance is the key to long-term success. As the Chinese say, a million is made up of nothing but lots of ones, and a bucket is quickly filled by steady drips and drops.

Exercise

Exercise is the second of what I call the three free therapies. According to Chinese medicine, regular and adequate exercise has two basic benefits. First, exercise promotes the movement of the qi and quickening of the blood. Since all IBS involves at least some component of liver depression qi stagnation, it is obvious that exercise is an important therapy for coursing the liver and rectifying the qi. Secondly, exercise benefits the spleen and therefore treats spleen qi vacuity, the other pattern which is always involved to some degree in IBS. The spleen's movement and transportation of the digestate is dependent upon the qi mechanism. The qi mechanism describes the function of the qi in upbearing the pure and downbearing the turbid parts of digestion. For the qi mechanism to function properly, the qi must be flowing normally and freely. Since exercise moves and rectifies the qi, it also helps regulate and rectify the qi mechanism. This then results in the spleen's movement and transportation of foods and liquids and its subsequent engendering and transforming of the qi and blood. In addition, a healthy spleen checks and controls a depressed liver. Therefore, it is easy to see that regular, adequate exercise is a vitally important component of any regime for either preventing or treating IBS.

What kind of exercise is best for IBS?

In my experience, I find aerobic exercise to be the most beneficial for most people with IBS. By aerobic exercise, I mean any physical activity which raises one's heartbeat 80% above their normal resting rate and keeps it there for at least 20 minutes. To calculate your normal resting heart rate, place your fingers over the pulsing artery on the front side of your neck. Count the beats for 15 seconds and then multiply by four. This gives you your beats per minute or BPM. Now multiply your BPM by 0.8. Take the resulting number and add it to your resting BPM. This gives you your aerobic threshold of BPM. Next engage in any physical activity you like. After you have been exercising for five minutes, take your pulse for 15 seconds once again at the artery on the front side of your throat. Again multiply the resulting count by four and this tells you your current BPM. If this number is less than your aerobic threshold BPM, then you know you need to exercise harder or faster. Once you get your heart rate up to your aerobic threshold, then you need to keep exercising at the same level of intensity for at least 20 minutes. In order to insure that one is keeping their heartbeat high enough for long enough, one should recount their pulse every five minutes or so.

Depending on one's age and physical condition, different people will have to exercise harder to reach their aerobic threshold than others. For some, simply walking briskly will raise their heartbeat 80% above their resting rate. For others, they will need to do calisthenics, running, swimming, racquetball, or some other, more strenuous exercise. It really does not matter what the exercise is as long as it raises your heartbeat 80% above your resting rate and keeps it there for 20 minutes. However, there are two other criteria that should be met. One, the exercise should be something that is not too boring. If it is too boring, then you may have a hard time keeping up your schedule. Since most people do find aerobic exercises such as running, stationary bicycles, and stair-steppers boring, it is good to listen to music or watch TV in order to distract your mind from the tedium. Secondly, the type of exercise should not cause any damage to any parts of the body. For instance, running on pavement may cause knee problems for some people. Therefore, you should pick a type of exercise you enjoy but also one which will not cause any problems.

When doing aerobic exercise, it is best to exercise either every day or every other day. If one does not do their aerobics at least once every 72 hours, then its cumulative effects will not be as great. Therefore, I recommend that my IBS patients do some sort of aerobic exercises every day or every other day, three to four times per week *at least*. The good news is that there is no real need to exercise more than 30 minutes at any one time. Forty-five minutes per session is not going to be all that much better than 25 minutes per session. And 25 minutes four times per week is much better than one hour once a week.

Deep relaxation

As we have seen above, IBS is associated with liver depression qi stagnation. In Chinese medicine, liver depression comes from not fulfilling all one's desires. But as we have also seen above, no adult can fulfill all their desires. This is why a certain amount of liver depression is endemic among adults. When our desires are frustrated, our qi becomes depressed. This then creates emotional depression and easy anger or irritability. In Chinese medicine, anger is nothing other than the venting of pent up qi in the liver. When qi becomes depressed in the liver, it accumulates like hot air in a balloon. Eventually, that hot, depressed, angry qi has to go somewhere. So when there is a little more frustration or stress, then this angry qi in the liver may vent itself upward as irritability, anger, shouting, or nasty words. Or the accumulated qi may vent sideways to the spleen and stomach and manifest as abdominal pain, cramping, constipation or diarrhea.

Essentially, this type of anger and irritability are due to a maladaptive coping response that is typically learned at a young age. When we feel frustrated or stressed, stymied by or angry about something, most of us tense our muscles and especially the muscles in our upper back and shoulders, neck, and jaws. At the same time, many of us will hold our breath. In Chinese medicine, the sinews are governed by the liver. This tensing of the muscles, *i.e.*, the sinews, constricts the flow of qi in the channels and network vessels. Since it is the liver which is responsible for the coursing and discharging of this qi, such tensing of the sinews leads to liver depression qi stagnation. Because the lungs govern the downward spreading and movement of the qi, holding our breath due to stress or frustration only worsen this tendency of the qi not to move and, therefore, to become depressed in the Chinese medical idea of the liver.

Therefore, deep relaxation is the third of the three free therapies. For deep relaxation to be therapeutic medically, it needs to be more than just mental equilibrium. It needs to be somatic or bodily relaxation as well as mental repose. Most of us no longer recognize that every thought we think and feeling we feel is actually a felt physical sensation somewhere in our body. The words we use to describe emotions are all abstract nouns, such as anger, depression, sadness, and melancholy. However, in Chinese medicine, *every emotion is associated with a change in the direction or flow of qi.* For instance, anger makes the qi move upward, while fear makes it move downward. Therefore, anger "makes our gorge rise" or "blow our top", while fear may cause a "sinking feeling" or make us "pee in our pants." These colloquial expressions are all based on the age-old wisdom that all thoughts and emotions are not just mental but also bodily events. This is why it is not just enough to clear one's mind. Clearing one's mind is good, but for really marked therapeutic results, it is even better if one clears one's mind at the same time as relaxing every muscle in the body as well as the breath.

Guided deep relaxation tapes

The single most efficient and effective way I have found for myself and my patients to practice such mental and physical deep relaxation is to do a daily, guided, progressive, deep relaxation audiotape. What I mean by guided is that a narrator on the tape leads one through the process of deep relaxation. Such tapes are progressive since they lead one through the body in a progressive manner, first relaxing one body part and then moving on to another. For instance, the narrator may say something to the effect that, as you exhale, you should feel your forehead get heavy and relaxed, softening and expanding, becoming warm and heavy. As you exhale again, now feel your cheeks get heavy and relaxed, softening and expanding, becoming warm and heavy. Breathe in and breathe out, letting your breath go without hindrance or hesitation. Breathing out, now feel your jaw muscles become heavy and relaxed, expanding and softening, becoming warm and heavy, etc., etc. throughout the entire body until one comes to the bottoms of one's feet.

There are innumerable such tapes on the market. These are usually sold in health food stores, New Age music and supply stores, or in bookstores with a good selection of New Age books. Over the years of suggesting this method of deep relaxation to my patients, I have found that each patient will have his or her own preferences in terms of the type of voice, male or female, the choice of words and imagery, whether there is background music or not, and the actual pace of the progression through the body. Therefore, I suggest listening to and even purchasing more than one such tape. One should find a tape which they like and can listen to without internal criticism or comment, going along like a cloud in the sky as the narrator's voice blows away all your mental and bodily stress and tension. If one has more than one tape, one can also switch every now and again from tape to tape so as not to become bored with the process or desensitized to the instructions.

Key things to look for in a good relaxation tape

In order to get the full therapeutic effect of such deep relaxation tapes, there are several key things to check for. First, be sure that the tape is a guided tape and not a subliminal relaxation tape. Subliminal tapes usually have music and any instructions to relax are given so quietly that they are not consciously heard. Although such tapes can help you feel relaxed when you do them, ultimately they do not teach you how to relax as a skill which can be consciously practiced and refined. Secondly, make sure the tape starts from the top of the body and works downward. Remember, anger makes the qi go upward in the body, and people with IBS due to liver depression qi stagnation already have too much qi rising upward in their bodies and becoming stagnant in their abdomens. Such depressed qi typically needs not only to be moved but also downborne. Third, make sure the tape instructs you to relax your physical body. If you do not relax all your muscles or sinews, the qi cannot flow freely and the liver cannot be coursed. Depression is not resolved, and there will not be the same medically therapeutic effect. And lastly, be sure the tape instructs you to let your breath go with each exhalation. One of the symptoms of liver depression is a stuffy feeling in the chest which we then unconsciously try to relieve by sighing. Letting each exhalation go completely helps the lungs push the qi downward. This allows the lungs to control the liver at the same time as it downbears upwardly counterflowing angry liver qi.

The importance of daily practice

In Shanghai in the People's Republic of China, there is a hospital where they use deep relaxation as a therapy with patients with high blood pressure, heart disease, stroke, and migraines. Research at this hospital shows how such daily, progressive deep relaxation can regulate the blood pressure and body temperature and improve the appetite, digestion, elimination, sleep, energy, and mood. One of the things they say at this hospital is, "Small results in 100 days, big results in 1,000." This means that if one does such daily, progressive deep relaxation *every single day for 100 days*, one will definitely experience certain results. What are these "small" results? These small results are improvements in all the parameters listed above: blood pressure, body temperature, appetite, digestion, elimination, sleep, energy, and mood. If these are "small" results, then what are the "big" results experienced in 1,000 days of practice? The "big" results are a change in how one reacts to stress—in other words, a change in one's very personality or character.

What these doctors in Shanghai stressed and what I have also experienced both personally and with my patients is that it is vitally important to do such daily, guided, progressive deep relaxation every single day, day in and day out for a solid three months at least and for a continuous three years at best. If you do such progressive, somatic deep relaxation every day, you will see every parameter or measurement of health and well-being improve. If you do this kind of deep relaxation only sporadically, missing a day here and there, it will feel good when you do it, but it will not have the marked, cumulative therapeutic effects it can. Therefore, perseverance is the real key to getting the benefits of deep relaxation.

The real test

Doing such a daily deep relaxation regime is like hitting tennis balls against a wall or hitting a bucket of balls at a driving range.

It is only practice; it is not the real game itself. A daily deep relaxation regime is done not only in order to relieve one's immediate stress and strain. It is done to learn a new skill, a new way to react to stress. The ultimate goal is to learn how to breathe out and immediately relax all one's muscles in the body in reaction to stress, rather than the common but unhealthy maladaption to stress of holding one's breath and tensing one's muscles. By doing such deep relaxation day after day, you will learn how to relax any and every muscle in your body quickly and efficiently. Then, as soon as you recognize that you are feeling frustrated, stressed out, or uptight, you can immediately remedy those feelings at the same time as coursing your liver and rectifying your qi. This is the real test, the game of life. "Small results in 100 days, big results in 1,000."

Finding the time

If you're like me and most of my patients, you are probably asking yourself right now, "All this is well and good, but when am I supposed to find the time to eat well-balanced cooked meals, exercise at least every other day, and do a deep relaxation every day? I'm already stretched to the breaking point." I know. That's the problem.

As a clinician, I often wish I could wave a magic wand over my patients' heads and make them all healthy and well. I cannot. After close to two decades of working with thousands of patients, I know of no easy way to health. There is good living and there is easy living. Or perhaps I am stating this all wrong. What most people take as the easy way these days is to continue pushing their limits continually to the max. The so-called path of least resistance is actually the path of lots and lots of resistance. Unless you take time for yourself and find the time to eat well, exercise, and relax, no treatment is going to eliminate your IBS completely. There is simply no pill you can pop or food you can eat that will get rid of the root causes of IBS: poor diet, too little exercise, and too much stress. Even Chinese herbal medicine and acupuncture can only get their full effect if the diet and lifestyle is first adjusted. Sun Si-maio, the most famous Chinese doctor of the Tang dynasty (618-907 CE), who himself refused government office and lived to be 101, said: "First adjust the diet and lifestyle and only secondarily give herbs and acupuncture." Likewise, it is said today in China, "Three parts treatment, seven parts nursing." This means that any cure is only 30% due to medical treatment and 70% is due to nursing, meaning proper diet and lifestyle.

In my experience, this is absolutely true. Seventy percent of all disease will improve after three months of proper diet, exercise, relaxation, and lifestyle modification. Seventy percent! Each of us has certain nondiscretionary rituals we perform each day. For instance, you may always and without exception find the time to brush your teeth. Perhaps it is always finding the time to shower. For others, it may be always finding the time each day to eat lunch. And for 99.99% of us, we find time, no, we make the time to get dressed each day. The same applies to good eating, exercise, and deep relaxation. Where there's a will there's a way. If your IBS is bad enough, you can find the time to eat well, get proper exercise, and do a daily deep relaxation tape.

The solution to IBS is in your hands

Bob Flaws, a famous Chinese medical practitioner in Boulder, CO, likes to tell the story about his sojourns on the walking mall in the center of that town. On summer evenings, he and his wife often walk down this mall. Having treated so many patients over the years, it is not unusual for him to meet former patients on these strolls. Frequently, these patients begin by telling him they're sorry they haven't been in to see him in such a long time. They usually say this apologetically as if they have done something wrong. Bob then usually asks them how they've been. Often they tell him: "When my such-and-such flares up, I remember what you told me about my diet, exercise, and lifestyle. I then go back to doing my exercise or deep relaxation or I change my diet, and then my symptoms go away. That's why I haven't been in. I'm sorry."

However, such patients have no need to be sorry. This kind of story is music to a Chinese doctor's ears. When Bob hears that these patients are now able to control their own conditions by following the dietary and lifestyle advice he gave them, he knows that, as a Chinese doctor, he has done his job correctly. In Chinese medicine, the inferior doctor treats disease after it has appeared. The superior doctor prevents disease before it has arisen. If Bob and I can teach our patients how to cure their symptoms themselves by making changes in their diet and lifestyle, then we're approaching the goal of the high class Chinese doctor—the prevention of disease through patient education.

To get these kinds of benefits, however, one must make the necessary changes in eating and behavior. In addition, IBS is not a condition that is cured once and forever like measles or mumps. When I say Chinese medicine can cure IBS, I do not mean that you will never experience symptoms again. What I mean is that Chinese medicine can eliminate or greatly reduce your symptoms *as long as you keep your diet and lifestyle together*. People being people, we all "fall off the wagon" from time to time and we all "choose our own poisons." I do not expect perfection from either my patients or myself. Therefore, I am not looking for a lifetime cure. Rather, I try to give my patients an understanding of what causes their disease and what they can do to minimize or eliminate its causes and mechanisms. It is then up to the patient to decide what is bearable and what is unbearable or what is an acceptable level of health. The Chinese doctor will have done their job when *you know how to correct your health to the level you find acceptable given the price you have to pay.*

9 Simple Home Remedies for IBS

Although faulty diet, lack of adequate exercise, and too much stress are the ultimate causes of IBS according to Chinese medicine and, therefore, diet, exercise, and deep relaxation are the most important in the treatment and prevention of IBS, there are a number of simple Chinese home remedies to help relieve the symptoms of IBS.

Chinese aromatherapy

In Chinese medicine, the qi is seen as a type of wind or vapor. The Chinese character for qi shows wind blowing over a rice field. In addition, smells are often referred to as a thing's qi. Therefore, there is a close relationship between smells carried through the air and the flow of qi in a person's body. Although aromatherapy has not been a major part of professionally practiced Chinese medicine for almost a thousand years, there is a simple aromatherapy treatment which one can do at home which can help alleviate irritability, depression, nervousness, anxiety, and insomnia.

In Chinese, *chen xiang* means "sinking fragrance." It is the name of Lignum Aquilariae Agallochae or Eaglewood. This is a frequent ingredient in Asian incense formulas. In Chinese medicine, Aquilaria is classified as a qi-rectifying medicinal. When used as a boiled decoction or "tea", Aquilaria moves the qi and stops pain, downbears upward counterflow and regulates the middle (*i.e.*, the spleen and stomach), and promotes the kidneys' grasping of the qi sent down by the lungs. I believe that the word sinking in this herb's name refers to this medicinal's downbearing of upwardly counterflowing qi. Such upwardly counterflowing qi eventually must accumulate in the heart, disturbing and causing restlessness of the heart spirit. When this medicinal wood is burnt and its smoke is inhaled as a medicinal incense, its downbearing and spirit-calming function is emphasized.

One can buy Aquilaria or *Chen Xiang* from Chinese herb stores in Chinatowns, Japantowns, or Koreatowns in major urban areas. One can also buy it from Chinese medical practitioners who have their own pharmacies. It is best to use the powdered variety. However, powder may be made by putting a small piece of this aromatic wood in a coffee grinder. It is also OK to use small bits of the wood if powder is not available. Next one needs to buy a roll of incense charcoals. Place one charcoal in a nonflammable dish and light it with a match. Then sprinkle a few pinches of Aquilaria powder on the lit charcoal. As the smoke rises, breathe in deeply. This can be done on a regular basis one or more times per day or on an as-needed basis by those suffering from restlessness, nervousness, anxiety, irritability, and depression. For those who experience insomnia, one can do this "treatment" when lying in bed at night.

This Chinese aromatherapy with Lignum Aquilariae Agallochae is very cheap and effective. I know of no side effects or contraindications.

Light therapy

Light therapy, more specifically sunbathing or heliotherapy, is one of Chinese medicine's health preservation and longevity practices. Sunlight is considered the most essential yang qi in nature. Li Shi-zhen, one of the most famous Chinese doctors of the late Ming dynasty (1368-1644 CE) wrote, "*Tai yang* (literally, supreme yang but a name for the sun) is true fire." As he pointed out, "Without fire, heaven is not able to engender things, and without fire, people are not able to live." Because the back of the human body is yang (as compared to the front which is more yin), exposing the back to sunlight is a good way of increasing one's yang qi.

As we have seen above, most people's yang qi begins to decline by around 35 years of age. In those over 35 years of age loose stools, lack of strength, poor memory, lack of concentration, poor coordination, decline in or lack of libido, low back and knee soreness and weakness, increased nighttime urination, and cold hands and feet are mostly due to this decline first in the yang qi of the spleen and later in the yang qi of the spleen and kidneys. When some people say they are depressed, what they often mean in Chinese medical terms is that they are extremely fatigued. In such cases, sunbathing can help supplement the yang qi of the body, thereby strengthening the spleen and/or kidneys.

Furthermore, because the yang qi is also the motivating force which pushes the qi, increasing yang qi can also help resolve depression and move stagnation. Cao Ting-dong, a famous doctor of the Qing dynasty (1644-1911 CE) wrote:

> Sitting with the back exposed directly to the sun, the back may get warmed. This is able to make the entire body harmonious and smoothly flowing. The sun is the essence of *tai yang* and its light strengthens the yang qi of the human body.

In Chinese medicine, whenever the words harmonious and smoothly flowing are used together, they refer to the flow of qi and blood. Hence sunbathing can help course the liver and rectify the qi as well as fortify the spleen and invigorate the kidneys.

It has been said that sunlight is good for every disease except skin cancer. As we now know, overexposure to the sun can cause skin cancer due to sunlight damaging the cells of the skin. Therefore, one should be careful not to get too much sun and not to get burnt. In Chinese medicine, sunbathing should be done between the hours of 8-10 AM. One should only sunbathe between 11 AM-1 PM in winter in temperate, not tropical, latitudes.

Hydrotherapy

Hydrotherapy means water therapy and is a part of traditional Chinese medicine. There are numerous different water treatments for helping relieve various symptoms of IBS. First, let's begin with a warm bath. If one takes a warm bath just slightly higher than body temperature for 15-20 minutes, this can free and smooth the flow of qi and blood. In addition, it can calm the spirit and hasten sleep. Taking a warm bath a half hour before going to bed can help some types of insomnia. It can also relieve tension and irritability.

However, when using a warm bath, one must be careful not to use water so hot or to stay in the bath so long that sweat breaks out on one's forehead. We lose yang qi as well as body fluids when we sweat. Because "fluids and blood share a common source", excessive sweating can cause problems for those with blood and yin vacuities. Sweating can also worsen yang qi vacuities in people whose spleen and kidneys are weak. Therefore, unless one is given a specific hot bath prescription by their Chinese medical practitioner, I suggest those with IBS not stay in warm baths until they sweat. Although they may feel pleasantly relaxed, they may later feel excessively fatigued or excessively hot and thirsty.

If, due to depression transforming heat, yang qi is exuberant and counterflowing upward, it may cause tension headaches or extreme irritability. In this case, one can tread in cold water up to their ankles for 15-20 minutes at a time. One may also soak their hands in cold water. Or they may put cold, wet compresses on the backs of their necks. The first two treatments seek to draw yang qi away from the head to either the lower part of the body or out to the extremities. The third treatment seeks to block and neutralize yang qi from counterflowing upward, congesting in the head and damaging the blood vessels in the head.

For those who are struggling with obesity, one can use cool baths slightly lower than body temperature for 10 minutes per day.

Although this may seem contradictory, since cold is yin and these patients already suffer from a yang insufficiency, this brief and not too extreme exposure to cool water stimulates the body to produce more yang qi. In Chinese medicine, it is not thought advisable for women to take cold baths during menstruation as this may retard the free flow of qi and blood and lead to dysmenorrhea or painful menstruation.

For abdominal pain due to qi stagnation, one can apply warm, wet compresses to the abdomen for 15-20 minutes at a time. One should not sleep with a hot water bottle or heating pad. If one uses such a hot application for too long, it begins to raise the body temperature. The body must maintain its normal temperature of 98.6° F. Therefore, if the body temperature goes up due to local application of heat, the body's response is to actually cut off the blood flow to that area of the body. This then would result in just the opposite, unwanted effect. Cooking several slices of fresh ginger in the water at a low boil for five to seven minutes and then using the resulting "tea" to make the hot compress can increase the compresses effect of moving the qi.

Chinese self-massage

Massage, including self-massage, is a highly developed part of traditional Chinese medicine. At its most basic, rubbing promotes the flow of qi and blood in the area rubbed. Below are three Chinese self-massage regimes. The first is a general protocol for mental stress that can also be used if there is insomnia, mental fatigue or poor mental concentration, the second is for diarrhea, and the third is for constipation. In fact, there are Chinese self-massage regimes for many health problems such as headache, painful menstruation, nausea and vomiting, acne, all sorts of body pain, colds and flus, and dizziness. For more Chinese self-massage regimes, the reader should see Fan Ya-li's *Chinese Self-massage Therapy: The Easy Way to Health*, also published by Blue Poppy Press.

Self-massage for mental stress

Bai Hui (GV 20)

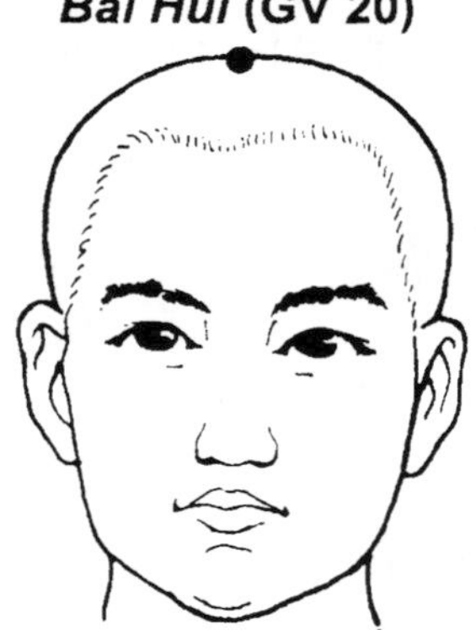

Begin by patting the top of the head with the hollow of the palm 20 times. The point in the middle of the top of the head is called *Bai Hui* (Meeting of Hundreds, Governing Vessel 20). Stimulation of this point calms the spirit and downbears upwardly counterflowing and exuberant liver yang. Do this 20 times.

Zan Zhu (Bl 2)

Next, use the tips of both index or middle fingers to press and knead the depression at the medial ends of the eyebrows (next to the nose) 30 times. This is the acupuncture point *Zan Zhu* (Bladder 2) which clears the head.

Third, bend the two index fingers and push with their radial (thumb) sides from the middle to the left and right sides of the forehead. Do this 20 times.

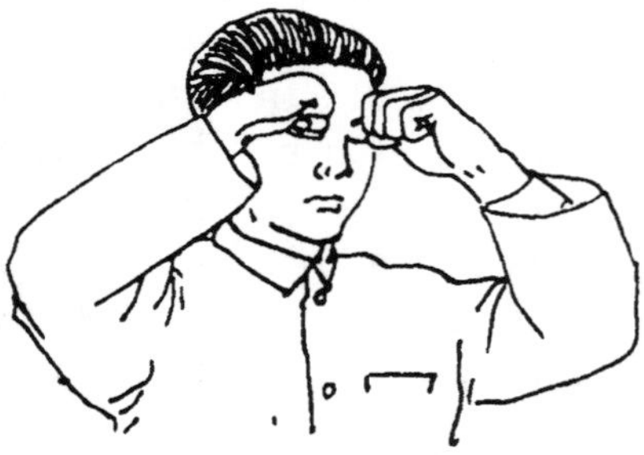

Fourth, on both sides of the head, find the spot where a line drawn horizontally half an inch above the front hairline and a line drawn vertically half an inch behind the hairline at the temple would meet. This is the point *Tou Wei* (Stomach 8). Press and knead 30 times.

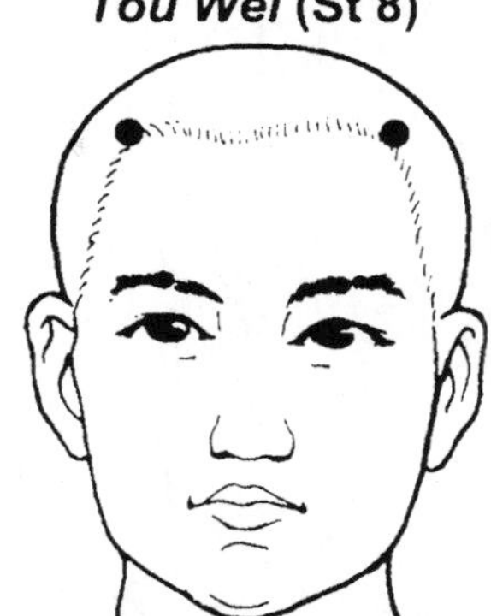

Fifth, press and knead the base of the skull in the depressions on both sides of the back of the neck 30 times. This is the acupuncture point *Feng Chi* (Gallbladder 20) and is a major point for treating upwardly counterflowing liver qi.

Sixth, press and knead the spot at the base of the skull at the midline 30 times. This point, *Feng Fu* (Governing Vessel 16), is for calming the spirit.

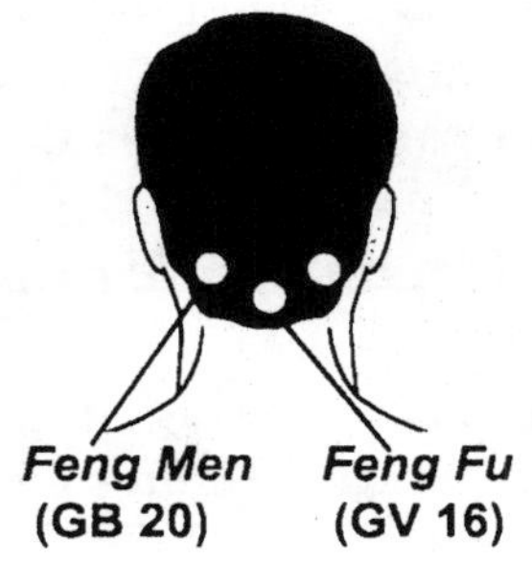

Seventh, press and knead *Shen Men* (Heart 7). This point is located on the inner wrist crease, just below the palm. As you are looking at your palm the point is on a line down from the little finger on the medial side of the tendon. This point also calms the spirit.

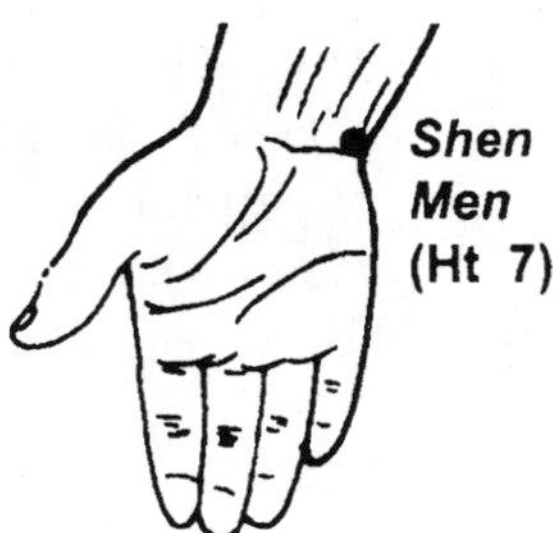

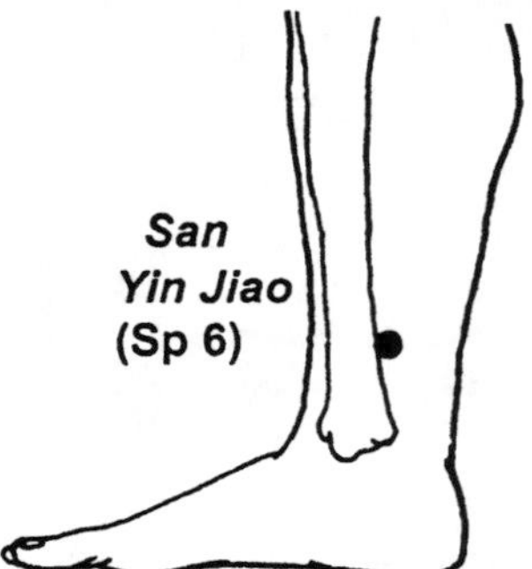

Eighth, press and knead *San Yin Jiao* (Spleen 6). This point is an intersection of the spleen, liver, and kidney channels. It supplements the spleen and stomach, harmonizes the liver, and calms the spirit. It is located three inches above the tip of the inner anklebone on the back edge of the tibia or lower leg bon

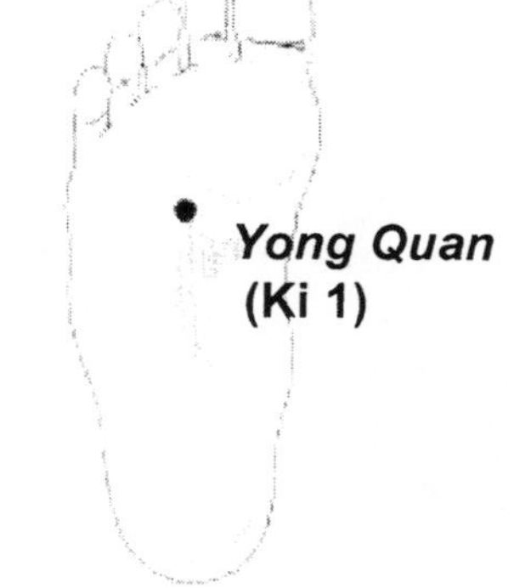

Finally, rub *Yong Quan* (Kidney 1) with a circular motion. This point is located on the bottom of the foot, approximately one third of the distance between the base of the second toe and the heel. *Yong Quan* supplements the kidneys, regulates the stool, calms the liver and rouses the brain.

Self-massage for chronic diarrhea

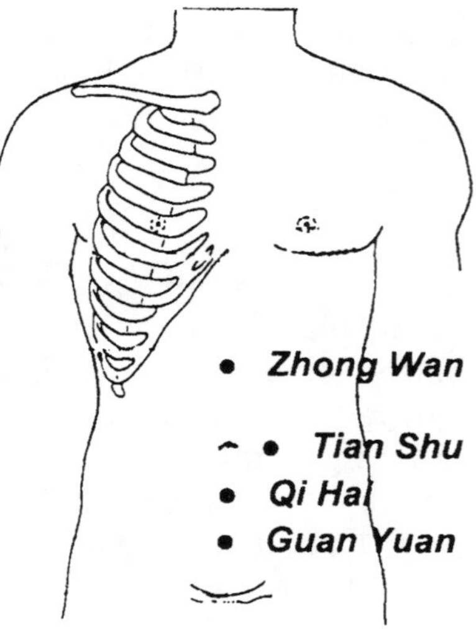

Begin by pressing and kneading four points 30 times each. First press and knead *Zhong Wan* (Conception Vessel 12). This point is located on the midline of the abdomen, halfway between the lower tip of the sternum and the navel. Next press and knead *Qi Hai* (Conception Vessel 6). This point is on the midline of the lower abdomen, two finger breadths below the navel. Then press and knead *Quan Yuan* (Conception Vessel 4). This point is located four finger breadths below the navel on the midline of the lower abdomen. Finally, press and knead *Tian Shu* (Stomach 25), which is located two inches from the center of the navel on both sides.

Conception Vessel 12 regulates the spleen and stomach, the root of qi and blood engenderment and transformation. Conception Vessel 6 regulates and fortifies the qi in the entire body. Conception Vessel 4 fortifies the spleen and nourishes the kidneys. Stomach 25 regulates the spleen, stomach and intestines and is indicated for digestive symptoms including diarrhea, constipation, poor appetite, abdominal pain, and rumbling intestines.

Next, use the first three fingers and rub the following two points in a counterclockwise direction, 50 times each. *Shen Que* (Conception Vessel 8) is located at the navel. *Dan Tian* (Cinnabar Field) is located three finger breadths directly below the navel.

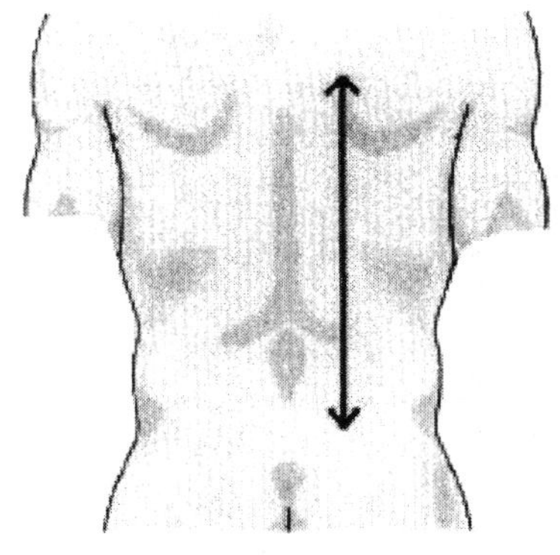

Third, press and knead all down the large muscles on either side of the spine. Press and knead approximately one and a half inches on either side of the spine. There are acupuncture points along the spine which connect directly with all the viscera and bowels. The production and function of the qi and blood is dependent on the proper functioning of the viscera and bowels.

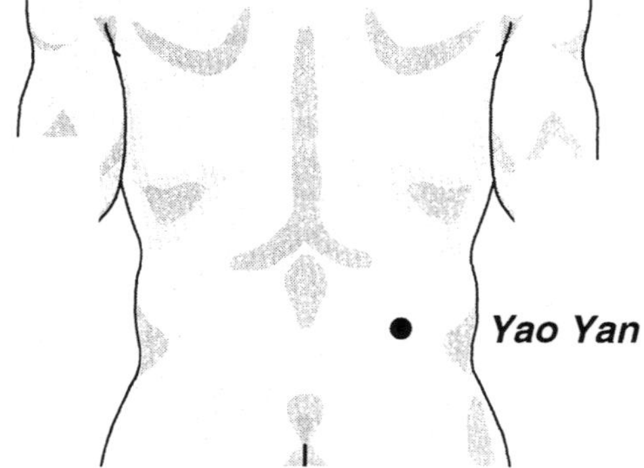

Fourth, make the hand into a loose fist and use the thumb side of the hand to scrub back and forth on the point *Yao Yan* (Eyes of the Lumbus, extra point M-BW-24). *Yao Yan* is located next to the fourth lumbar vertebra, approximately 3.5 inches to either side.

Fifth, scrub the low back or lumbosacral region. Scrub back and forth from side to side until the area becomes warm to the touch. "The low back is the mansion of the kidneys," and this stimulates the kidneys, remembering that sufficient kidney yang is necessary for normal functioning of the spleen and stomach.

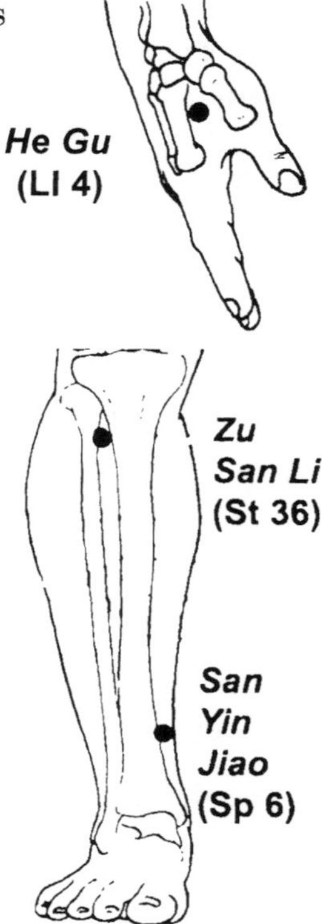

Last, press and knead three points 30 times each. The first point is *He Gu* (Large Intestine 4). Large Intestine 4 is located on the bulge of the muscle between the thumb and index finger when they are pressed together, press this point to the side against the first metacarpal bone in the hand. The second point is *Zu San Li* (Stomach 36). This point is located three inches below the lower, outside edge of the knee-cap. This point regulates the qi of the entire body, regulates the qi of the stomach channel in particular, and fortifies the spleen at the same time as it harmonizes the stomach. The third point is *San Yin Jiao* (Spleen 6). This point is an inter-section of the spleen, liver and kidney channels. It has many functions including supplementing the spleen and stomach, harmonizing the liver, nourishing the kidneys and calming the spirit. It is located three inches above the tip of the inner anklebone on the back edge of the tibia or lower leg bone.

If the diarrhea is worse with mental-emotional stress and is accompanied by abdominal pain, rumbling intestines or distention in the abdomen, ribside or chest, the following two points may be pressed and kneaded 30 times each.

First, press and knead *Nei Guan* (Pericardium 6). This point is located on the palmar side of the forearm, two inches from the wrist crease, between the two tendons. It rectifies the qi, downbears counterflow, harmonizes the stomach and stops pain.

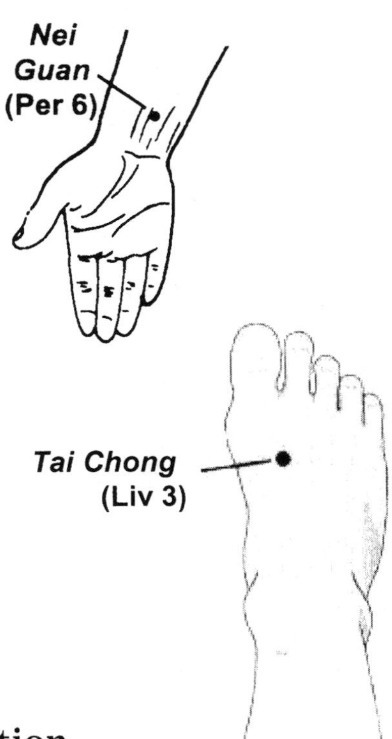

And finally, press and knead *Tai Chong* (Liver 3) to soothe the liver and rectify the qi. Liver 3 is on the top of the foot in the depression between the first and second metatarsal bones just distal to where the tarsal and metatarsal bones meet.

Self-massage for constipation

First, knead Stomach 25 and Conception Vessel 4, 30 times each. The locations of these points are given above in the first step of the self-massage protocol for diarrhea. Together these they fortify the spleen, nourish the kidneys and regulate the digestion.

Next, rub the lower abdomen clockwise 50 times.

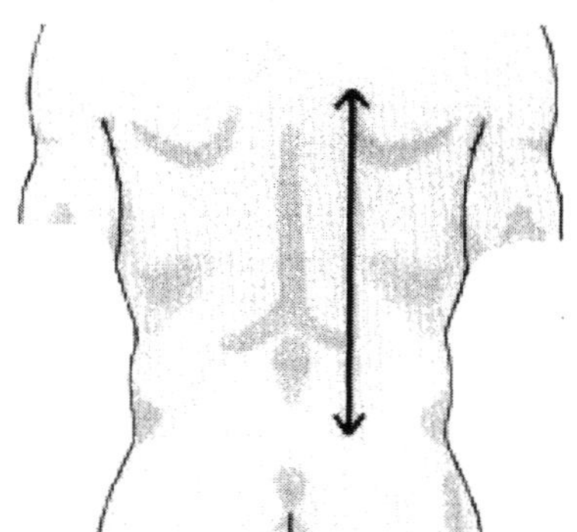

Third, press and knead all down the large muscles on either side of the spine. Press and knead approximately one and a half inches on either side of the spine. There are acupuncture points along the spine which connect directly with all the viscera and bowels. The production and function of the qi and blood is dependent on the proper functioning of the viscera and bowels.

Fourth, press and knead *Zhi Gou* (Triple Burner 6) 30 times. This point is located on the back of the arm, three inches from the wrist between the radius and the ulna (the two bones in the forearm). It clears the triple burner, frees the bowel qi and downbears counterflow qi and fire and is often used to treat constipation and abdominal pain.

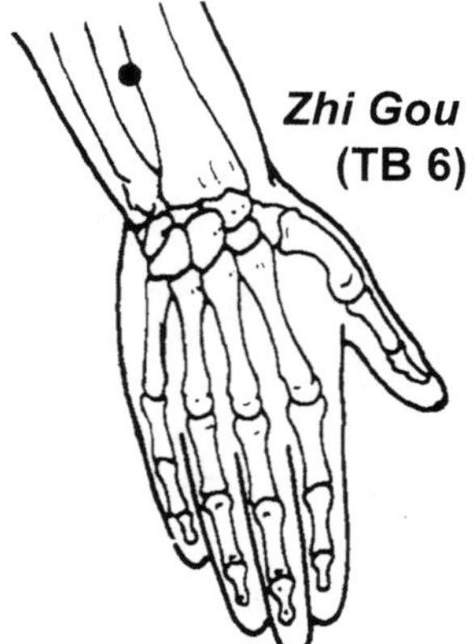

Fifth, press and knead, two points 30 times each. The first point is Large Intestine 4 and the second is Stomach 36. The locations of these two points are given under the last step of the self-massage protocol for diarrhea above. In this case, Large Intestine 4 is used to free gastrointestinal downbearing. Stomach 36 regulates the qi of the entire body, regulates the qi of the stomach channel in particular, and fortifies the spleen at the same time as it harmonizes the stomach.

Sixth, with the palms of the hands pat the side of the lower leg, from the knee to the ankle, 10 times on each leg.

Finally, grasp *Cheng Shan* (Bladder 57) 10 times. Bladder 57 is located on the back of the lower leg between the two heads of the gastrocnemius muscle. Grasping means to slowly lift, squeeze and knead the muscle with the thumb and index finger. Bladder 57 harmonizes the intestines and treats constipation.

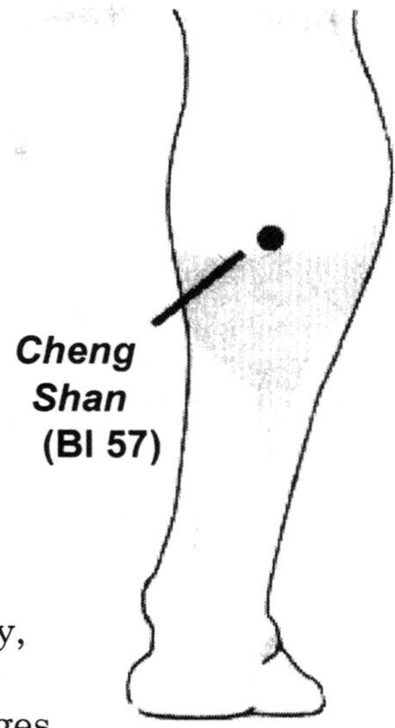

The key to success with Chinese self-massage therapy is perseverance. Although a single massage may provide some symptomatic relief on that very day, it is repeated self-massage day after day which can make stable and lasting changes.

Chinese foot therapy

Foot reflexology is also a part of contemporary Chinese medicine. Chinese doctors have adopted Western foot reflexology and added to it Chinese diagnosis and treatment protocols. According to foot reflexology theory, various areas on the bottoms of the feet correspond with various viscera and bowels in the body. By stimulating these areas on the feet, one can effect the function of the corresponding viscera and bowels. Usually the method of stimulation is a strong, kneading pressure on the associated areas to be treated. One can use either the ball of their thumb or the eraser on a pencil. Shops selling massage implements often have special wooden foot zone stimulators. In order to increase the circulation in the feet to make this therapy even more effective, one can soak the feet in warm or hot water prior to treatment.

Diarrhea

To treat diarrhea, strongly stimulate the following reflex zones on the bottoms of the feet: spleen, stomach, liver, ascending, transverse, and descending colon. Please note that, because the internal organs are not arranged symmetrically, the zones on the feet are also not bilaterally symmetrical. Treat one time per day during acute episodes and taper off as the diarrhea likewise recedes in severity.

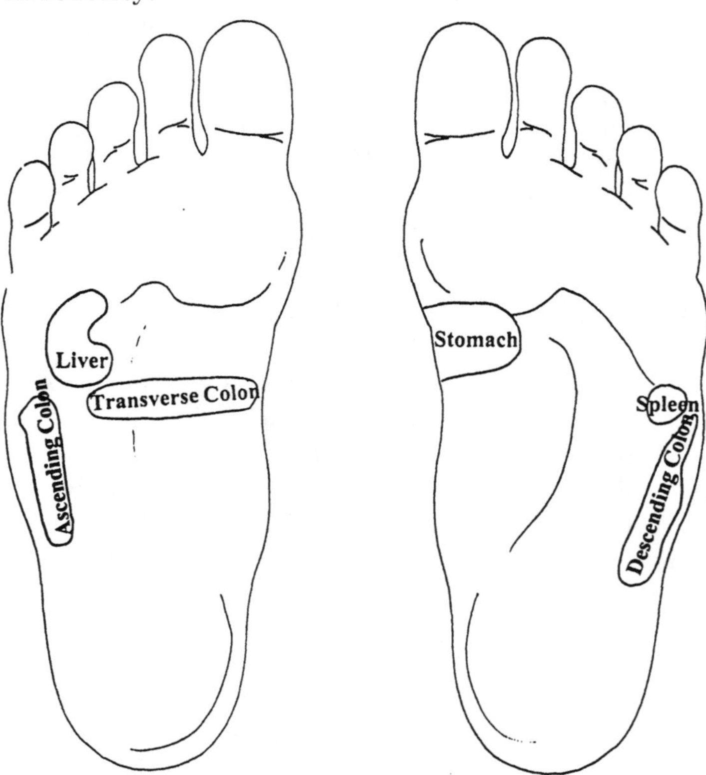

Constipation

For constipation, strongly stimulate the following foot reflex zones: rectum, anus, ascending, transverse, and descending colon. If there is liver depression qi stagnation, as there usually is in IBS, also stimulate the liver. If there is spleen vacuity, also stimulate the spleen. Treat one time per day or every other day.

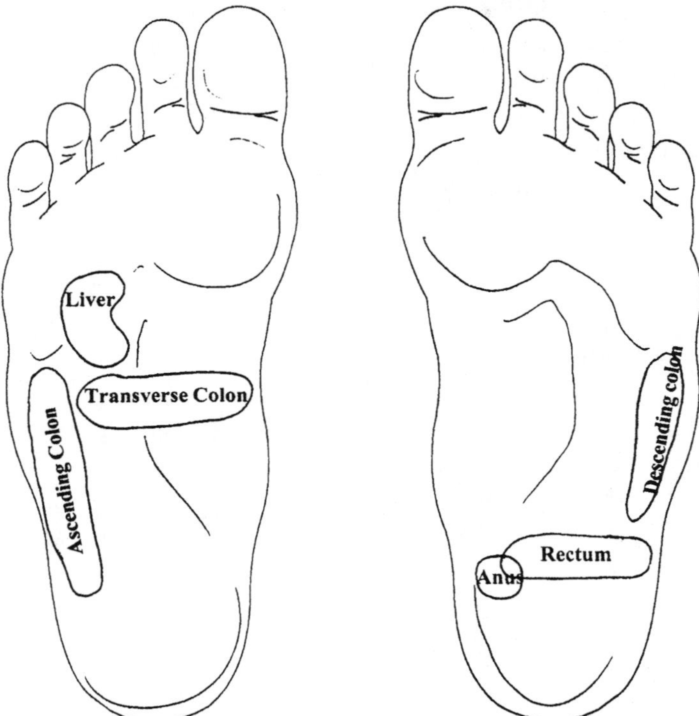

Flower therapy

People have been bringing other people flowers for millennia to help them feel good. In Chinese medicine, there is actually a practice of flower therapy. Because the beauty of flowers bring most people joy and because joy is the antidote to the other four or seven negative emotions of Chinese medicine, flowers can help promote the free and easy flow of qi. It is said in Chinese medicine that, "Joy leads to relaxation (in the flow of qi)", and relaxation is exactly what the doctor ordered in cases of liver depression qi stagnation. As Wu Shi-ji wrote in the Qing dynasty,

"Enjoying flowers can divert a person from their boredom and alleviate suffering caused by the seven affects (or emotions)."

However, there is more to Chinese flower therapy than the beauty of flowers bringing joy. Flower therapy also includes aromatherapy. A number of Chinese medicinals come from plants which have flowers used in bouquets. For instance, Chrysanthemum flowers (*Ju Hua*, Flos Chrysanthemi Morifolii) are used to calm the liver and clear depressive heat rising to the upper body. The aroma of Chrysanthemum flowers thus also has a salutary, relaxing, and cooling effect on liver depression and depressive heat. Rose (*Mei Gui Hua,* Flos Rosae Rugosae) is used in Chinese medicine to move the qi and quicken the blood. Smelling the fragrance of Roses also does these same things. Other flowers used in Chinese medicine to calm the spirit and relieve stress and irritability are Lily, Narcissus, Lotus flowers, Orchids, and Jasmine. And further, taking a smell of a bouquet of flowers promotes deep breathing, and this, in turn, relieves pent up qi in the chest at the same time as it promotes the flow of qi downward via the lungs.

Thread moxibustion

Thread moxibustion refers to burning extremely tiny cones or "threads" of aged Oriental mugwort directly on top of certain acupuncture points. When done correctly, this is a very simple and effective way of adding yang qi to the body without causing a burn or scar.

To do thread moxa, one must first purchase the finest grade Japanese moxa wool. This is available from Oriental Medical Supply Co. located at 1950 Washington St., Braintree, MA 02184; Tel: (617) 331-3370 or 800-323-1839; Fax: (617) 335-5779. It is listed under the name Gold Direct Moxa. Pinch off a very small amount of this loose moxa wool and roll it lightly between the thumb and forefinger. What you want to wind up with is a very loose, very thin thread of moxa smaller than a grain of rice. It is important that this thread not be too large or too tightly wrapped.

Next, rub a very thin film of Tiger Balm or Temple of Heaven Balm on the point to be moxaed. These are camphorated Chinese medical salves which are widely available in North American health food stores. Be sure to apply nothing more than the thinnest film of salve. If such a Chinese medicated salve is not available, then wipe the point with a tiny amount of vegetable oil. Stand the thread of moxa up perpendicularly directly over the point to be moxaed. The oil or balm should provide enough stickiness to make the thread stand on end. Light the thread with a burning incense stick. As the thread burns down towards the skin, you will feel more and more heat. Immediately remove the burning thread when you begin to feel the burning thread go from hot to too hot. *Do not burn yourself.* It is better to pull the thread off too soon than too late. In this case, more is not better than enough. (If you do burn yourself, apply some *Ching Wan Hong* ointment. This is a Chinese burn salve which is available at Chinese apothecaries and is truly wonderful for treating all sorts of burns. It should be in every home's medicine cabinet.)

Having removed the burning thread and extinguished it between your two fingers, repeat this process again. To make this process go faster and more efficiently, one can roll a number of threads before starting the treatment. Each time the thread burns down close to the skin, pinch it off the skin and extinguish it *before* it starts to burn you. If you do this correctly, your skin will get red and hot to the touch but you will not raise a blister. Because everyone's skin is different, the first time you do this, only start out with three or four threads. Each day, increase this number until you reach nine to twelve threads per treatment.

This treatment is especially effective for women in their late 30s and throughout their 40s and men over 50 whose spleen and kidney yang qi has already become weak and insufficient. Since this treatment actually adds yang qi to the body, this type of thread moxa fortifies the spleen and invigorates the kidneys, warming yang and boosting the qi. Because the stimuli is not that strong at any given treatment, it must be done every day for a number of days. For people who suffer from IBS with pronounced fatigue, loose stools, cold hands and feet, low or no libido, and low back or knee pain accompanied by frequent nighttime urination which tends to be copious and clear, I recommend that this moxibustion be done every day for a month, stopped for a week or so, and then repeated. It can be done for several months in a row, but should not usually be done continuously throughout the year, day in and day out. Whenever symptoms get better it means that the treatment is no longer needed and should be stopped.

There are three points which should be moxaed using this supplementing technique. These are:

Qi Hai (Conception Vessel 6)
Guan Yuan (Conception Vessel 4)
Zu San Li (Stomach 36)

We have already discussed how to locate these three points above (page 100-102). However, I recommend visiting a local professional acupuncturist so that they can teach you how to do this technique safely and effectively and to show you how to locate these three points accurately.

In Chinese medicine, this technique is considered a longevity and health preservation technique. It is great for those people whose yang qi has already begun to decline due to the inevitable aging process. It should not be done by people with ascension of hyperactive liver yang, liver fire, or depressive liver heat. It should also always be done starting from the topmost point and moving downward. This is to prevent leading heat to counterflow upward. If there is any doubt about whether this technique is appropriate for you, please see a professional practitioner for a diagnosis and individualized recommendation.

Magnet therapy

Magnet therapy means the treatment of various regions of the body by various sized and strengths of magnets. Although magnet therapy is currently experiencing something of a vogue here in the West, magnet therapy has been a part of traditional Chinese medicine since at least the Tang dynasty. Various sized self-adhesive magnets can be purchased from Oriental Medical Supplies Co. mentioned above under moxibustion.

Diarrhea & intestinal cramps

For diarrhea and intestinal cramps, choose from among *Zhong Wan* (Conception Vessel 12), *Shen Que* (Conception Vessel 8, the navel), *Tian Shu* (Stomach 25), *Zu San Li* (Stomach 36), *Da Chang Shu* (Bladder 25), and *Qi Hai* (Conception Vessel 6). The locations of all these points have been discussed above. Use 3-5 points each treatment, adhering the magnets with the south pole in touch with the skin. It is usually the south side of adhesive magnets that is already side up. Use small sized magnets on all these points except for Conception Vessel 12 and Conception Vessel 8 which typically require large or medium-sized ones. Leave in place for anywhere from several hours to a couple of days depending on the severity of the condition and the degree of relief obtained.

For diarrhea due to more pronounced spleen qi vacuity with marked fatigue and dizziness upon standing up, choose instead from: *Bai Hui* (Governing Vessel 20), *Qi Hai* (Conception Vessel 6), *Guan Yuan* (Conception Vessel 4), *Wei Shu* (Bladder 21), *Zu San Li* (Stomach 36), and *Zhong Wan* (Conception Vessel 12). Use 3-5 points per treatment and make sure the north side of the magnet is face down on the skin.

Constipation

For constipation due to either liver depression qi stagnation or heat in the stomach and intestines causing dry, hard, bound stools, choose from among *Zhong Wan* (Conception Vessel 12), *Tian Shu* (Stomach 25), *Zu San Li* (Stomach 36), *Qu Chi* (Large Intestine 11), and *Nei Ting* (Stomach 44), adhering the magnets with the south pole touching the skin. Use 3-5 points per treatment and leave in place for 2-3 days at a time. Large Intestine 11 is located at the end of the crease on the side of the elbow when it is flexed.

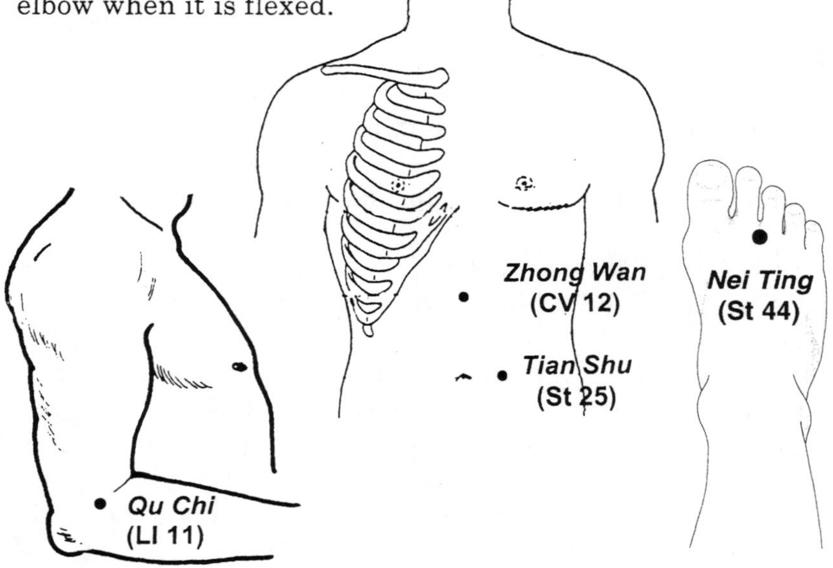

Stomach 44 is located at the end of the crease between the second and third toes on the top of the foot.

For more instructions on how you might incorporate magnet therapy into your self-care, see your local acupuncturist.

Chinese herbal teas

Although some people call professionally prescribed Chinese medicinal decoctions Chinese herbal teas, this name rightly belongs to simpler, one, two, and three ingredient teas which are either steeped or boiled. Typically, such Chinese medicinal teas can be drunk throughout the day as a background beverage and can greatly enhance the effects of acupuncture and other Chinese medicinal treatment with pills and powders. The ingredients in these teas can be purchased either at Oriental specialty food stores, your local Chinese medical practitioner, from Mayway Corp. and Nuherbs Co. listed in the chapter on Chinese herbal medicine, or from:

China Herb Co.
6333 Wayne Ave.
Philadelphia, PA 19144 USA
Tel: 215-843-5864 / 800-221-4372
Fax: 215-849-3338

Abdominal cramping & pain

Hyacinth bean tea (*Bian Dou Cha*)

This tea is suitable for damp heat in the stomach and intestines causing colicky pain which comes and goes and which may be associated with either diarrhea or constipation. This tea moves the qi and transforms dampness, clears heat and drains fire. It is made by pounding 30 fresh Semen Dolichoris Lablab (*Bai Bian Dou*) or hyacinth beans into a liquid. Place in a pot, add water, and bring to a boil. Drink frequently throughout the day as a tea.

Leechee nut tea (*Li Zhi He Cha*)

This tea is suitable for liver depression qi stagnation lower abdominal pain. It is made by placing 15 grams of Semen Litchi Chinensis (*Li Zhi He*) and 10 grams of Semen Citri Reticulatae

(*Ju He*) in a pot of water. Semen Citri Reticulatae are simply orange pits. Boil for 15 minutes at a medium heat. Then strain the liquid and drink freely as a tea.

Diarrhea

Plantain seed tea (*Che Qian Zi Cha*)

Stir-fry in a dry wok 10 grams of Semen Plantaginis (*Che Qian Zi*). Then steep these in boiling water with three grams of black tea. This tea is for spleen vacuity diarrhea complicated by dampness. Since spleen vacuity complicates most cases of IBS, this is generally a safe tea for most IBS sufferers to drink. It even helps against damp heat diarrhea. The above prescription is for one packet or dose, and you can drink this tea 2-3 times per day as long as you are not negatively effected by black tea.

Umeboshi & kudzu tea (*Wu Mei Ge Gen Cha*)

Place one fermented plum (called umeboshi in Japanese and *Wu Mei* in Chinese) and a teaspoon of kudzu or arrowroot powder in a cup of boiling water and stir till the kudzu powder is as dissolved as possible. One can also add a slice of fresh ginger to this if you want. That makes its ability to harmonize the qi and transform dampness stronger. Drink this tea several times per day. It is very effective for stopping diarrhea.

Treating dysentery rapidly & effectively tea (*Zhi Li Su Xiao Cha*)

This tea can treat damp heat, food stagnation, and qi stagnation types of diarrhea. It is made by first stir-frying nine grams of green tea leaves in a little salt water. When the leaves are dry, combine them with nine grams of Semen Arecae Catechu (*Bin Lang*) and water in a pot. Bring to a boil and allow to steep for 10 minutes. Drink this recipe warm 2-3 times per day.

Constipation

Senna leaf tea (*Fan Xie Ye Cha*)

Senna leaves are used in Chinese medicine just the same as in Western herbalism. For heat in the stomach and intestines causing dry, hard, bound stools, steep 1-3 grams of senna leaves in boiling water. Drink this frequently as a tea.

Contraindications: Senna is a purgative and has strong laxative action that may cause abdominal pain if the dose is too strong or it is not truly appropriate. It is contraindicated during pregnancy, for nursing mothers, during menstruation, and in individuals who are vacuous and weak. It is also not suitable for long-term use.

Sesame oil & honey tea (*Xiang Mi Cha*)

This tea is for dry stools constipation due to blood vacuity and large intestine fluid dryness. Add 65 grams of honey to 35 milliliters of roasted sesame oil. Roasted sesame oil can be found in the Oriental food section of most large Western grocery food stores. Pour this mixture into boiling water and stir. Take once in the morning and once in the evening.

Biota seed & honey tea (*Bai Ren Mi Cha*)

This tea is also for dry stools constipation due to blood and fluid vacuity. Grind 15 grams of Semen Biotae Orientalis (*Bai Zi Ren*) and boil with water. Then add honey to taste and drink 1-2 times per day. This tea moistens the intestines and frees the flow of the stools, quiets the heart and aids sleep. It is indicated for habitual constipation, typically in the elderly, accompanied by heart palpitations and/or insomnia due to yin vacuity and fluid dryness.

For more information on Chinese medicinal teas, see *Chinese Medicinal Teas: Simple, Proven, Folk Formulas for Common*

Diseases & Promoting Health by Zong Xiao-fang and Gary Liscum, available from Blue Poppy Press.

Chinese herbal porridges

Sometimes referred to as congee, there is a long history in Chinese medicine of combining one or two herbs with various types of porridge for the treatment and prevention of disease. There are literally hundreds of such medicinal porridge recipes in the Chinese medical literature. Chinese herbal porridges are especially useful for the treatment of all types of diarrhea and constipation. The ingredients for these porridges can be obtained from the same sources and suppliers as the Chinese herbal teas discussed above.

Diarrhea

Kudzu & rice porridge (*Ge Gen Fen Zhou*)

This porridge is good for spleen vacuity and damp heat types of diarrhea. It is made by cooking 30 grams of powdered kudzu or arrowroot in 50 grams of rice in a quart of water for several hours at a low boil. Once cooked, it can be eaten warm several times per day.

Chinese yam & egg yolk porridge (*Shan Yao Ji Zi Zhou*)

This porridge is for enduring diarrhea of many days duration due to primarily spleen vacuity. It is made by first powdering 50 grams of Radix Dioscoreae Oppositae (*Shan Yao*). Add water to form a thin gruel and bring to a boil 2-3 times. Then add and stir in the egg yolks. Eat this three times per day on an empty stomach.

Chinese yam & plantain seed porridge (*Shan Yao Che Qian Zi Zhou*)

Powder 30 grams of Radix Dioscoreae Oppositae (*Shan Yao*), add water, and stir into a thin gruel. Then add 12 grams of Semen Plantaginis (*Che Qian Zi*) wrapped in cheesecloth or a small cotton bag. Cook the resulting mixture into porridge and eat several times per day. It treats spleen vacuity with dampness and even some damp heat.

Cardamon porridge (*Bai Dou Kou Zhou*)

This porridge is for liver-spleen disharmony diarrhea with dampness. To make it, first cook 50 grams of rice in a quart of water into a thin porridge or gruel. During the last five minutes of cooking, add five grams of powdered cardamon. Eat this three times per day (along with other foods).

Constipation

Prune seed porridge (*Yu Li Ren Zhou*)

Soak five grams of prune seeds and remove the skins. Then mash into a paste. Cook 50 grams of rice into porridge with a quart of water. Then add the mashed prune seeds, a suitable amount of honey, and a little ginger juice. Eat on an empty stomach. This porridge is for the treatment of both qi stagnation and intestinal dryness constipation.

Pine nut porridge (*Song Ren Zhou*)

Cook 50 grams of rice and 30 grams of pine nuts in one quart of water into porridge. Add a suitable amount of honey at the end and eat two times per day on an empty stomach. This porridge treats fluid dryness constipation with hard, dry, bound stools.

For numerous other Chinese herbal porridge recipes, see Bob Flaws's *The Book of Jook: Chinese Medicinal Porridges, A Healthy Alternative to the Typical Western Breakfast* also available from Blue Poppy Press.

10
Chinese Medical Research on IBS

Considerable research has been done in the People's Republic of China on the effects of acupuncture and Chinese herbal medicine on all aspects of IBS. Usually, this research is in the form of a clinical audit. That means that a group of patients with the same diseases, patterns, or major complaints are given the same treatment for a certain period of time. After this time, the patients are counted to see how many were cured, how many got a marked effect, how many got some effect, and how many got no effect. This kind of "outcome-based research" has, up until only very recently, not been considered credible in the West where, for the last 30 years or so, the double-blind, placebo-controlled comparison study has been considered the "gold standard." However, such double-blind, placebo-controlled comparison studies are impossible to design in Chinese medicine and do not, in any case, measure effectiveness in a real-life situation.

Clinical audits, on the other hand, do measure actual clinical satisfaction of real-life patients. Such clinical audits may not exclude the patient's trust and belief in the therapist or the therapy as an important component in the result. However, real-life is not as neat and discreet as a controlled laboratory experiment. If the majority of patients are satisfied with the results of a particular treatment and there are no adverse side effects to that treatment, then that is good enough for the Chinese doctor, and, in my experience, that is also good enough for the vast majority of my patients.

Below are abbreviated translations of several recent research articles published in Chinese medical journals on the treatment of irritable bowel syndrome. These research articles are typical of how Chinese medicine treats IBS. I think that most people reading these statistics would think that Chinese medicine was worth a try. Therefore, below are some abstracts of recent Chinese medical journal articles describing the treatment of IBS with Chinese herbal medicine. I present this research for those readers who need "proof" that Chinese medicine does treat IBS effectively.

"The Treatment of 120 Cases of Irritable Bowel Syndrome Using *Shan Yao Che Qian Zi Tang* (Dioscorea & Plantaginis Decoction)," Chen Wei-di, *Shang Hai Zhong Yi Yao Za Zhi (Shanghai Journal of Chinese Medicine & Medicinals)*, #3, 1992, p. 33

In 1986, 120 patients were selected from a nationwide study of chronic diarrhea due to irritable bowel syndrome. There were 49 males and 71 females. The youngest participant was 18 years of age and the oldest was 53 years of age, with a median age of 36.4 years. The course of the illness ranged from 1 year and 1 month to 12 years, with the median duration of illness being 5 years and 1 month. One hundred eighteen patients had abdominal pain and 120 had diarrhea. Lab tests: 84 patients had mucus in their stools, 4 patients had a small amount of red blood cells in their stools and 28 had white blood cells in their stool culture. Fiber optic gastroscopy revealed slight edema in 32 cases, intestinal spasm in 7 cases, and an increase in intestinal mucosa in 66 cases. There was no incidence of organic pathological changes.

Seventy-eight patients had a Chinese medical differential diagnosis of liver depression and spleen vacuity. The symptoms defining this pattern were abdominal pain and diarrhea related to emotional upset. When the abdominal pain had persisted for a long time, there was an urge to have diarrhea after which the pain diminished. Accompanying this was thoracic oppression, a propensity to sigh, postprandial abdominal distention, depression, a propensity to become easily angered, soft stools, and flatulence. The tongue coating was either white or white and slimy, and the pulse was wiry. Forty-two patients conformed to a spleen-stomach vacuity pattern. There were symptoms of pasty diarrhea and a tendency to incautious eating, thus leading to an increased number of bowel movements, mucus, abdominal pain and distention, poor appetite, a pale, lusterless facial complexion, fatigued essence spirit, a pale tongue with a white coating, and a fine, weak pulse.

The primary prescription was Zhang Xi-chun's *Shan Yao Che Qian Zi Tang*: Radix Dioscoreae Oppositae (*Shan Yao*), 50g, and Semen Plantaginis (*Che Qian Zi*), 20g. The above two ingredients were cooked together into a thick porridge which was administered 3 times daily.

Once the diarrhea subsided the above prescription was administered with *Tong Xie Yao Fang* (Painful Diarrhea Essential Formula). This prescription then consisted of: Radix Dioscoreae Oppositae (*Shan Yao*), 12g, Semen Plantaginis (*Che Qian Zi*), 20g, Rhizoma Atractylodis Macrocephalae (*Bai Zhu*), 18g, Radix Albus Paeoniae Lactiflorae (*Bai Shao*), 15g, and Pericarpium Citri Reticulatae (*Chen Pi*), 12g.

If there was spleen-stomach vacuity, the following medicinals were added: Radix Astragali Membranacei (*Huang Qi*), Radix Codonopsitis Pilosulae (*Dang Shen*), Sclerotium Poriae Cocos (*Fu Ling*), and mix-fried Radix Glycyrrhizae (*Gan Cao*). If there was severe abdominal pain, the dose of Radix Albus Paeoniae Lactiflorae was doubled and Rhizoma Cyperi Rotundi (*Xiang Fu*) and Rhizoma Corydalis Yanhusuo (*Yan Hu Suo*) were added. If there was severe abdominal distention, Fructus Amomi (*Sha Ren*) and Semen Raphani Sativi (*Lai Fu Zi*) were added. If there was poor appetite, Massa Medica Fermentata (*Shen Qu*), Fructus Germinatus Hordei Vulgaris (*Mai Ya*), and Fructus Germinatus

Oryzae Sativae (*Gu Ya*) were added. This preparation was decocted in water and one packet was administered in two daily doses.

Eighty-one cases (67.5%) achieved a complete cure. This was defined as the disappearance of all clinical symptoms and either 1-2 bowel movements per day or a well-formed stool every other day. Laboratory tests revealed no mucus or red or white blood cells. Gastroscopy revealed decreased intestinal mucus and the disappearance of intestinal spasm. After one year, there was no recurrence of symptoms. Thirty-one cases (28.3%) achieved a good result. This meant that their clinical symptoms disappeared. Stools were frequent but, fundamentally, bowel movements were normal. The stools were a bit soft and there was still a small amount of mucus. After six months, there was no obvious relapse. Five cases (4.2%) experienced no clinical relief or experienced slight relief and then relapsed. Neither laboratory tests nor gastroscopy showed any appreciable changes.

Fifty-one cases (out of a possible 78 cases) falling into the liver depression-spleen vacuity pattern achieved a cure which took an average of 24 packets. Thirty cases (out of a possible 42) who exhibited the spleen-stomach vacuity pattern achieved a cure, taking an average of 26 packets.

"The Treatment of 33 Cases of Irritable Bowel Syndrome with *Tong Xie Yao Fang* (Painful Diarrhea Essential Formula)" by Yin Wei-che *et al.*, *Xin Zhong Yi (New Chinese Medicine)*, #3, 1998, p. 49

Beginning in 1984, the authors treated 33 cases of irritable bowel syndrome with *Tong Xie Yao Fang* and compared their outcomes with those of a comparison group treated with Western medicine.

The 57 patients in this study all had abdominal pain, abdominal distention, diarrhea, and constipation as their main symptoms. Based on diagnostic criteria developed at the 1996 Chinese

National Symposium on Chronic Diarrhea, all were diagnosed with irritable bowel syndrome. There were 26 men and 31 women ranging in age from 19-76 years old. Their course of disease ranged from three months to 12 years. In terms of sex, age, and disease duration, the 57 patients were divided into two groups which were statistically the same. There were 33 in the treatment group and 24 in the comparison group.

The treatment group was administered *Tong Xie Yao Fang* as their basic formula. It was composed of: stir-fried Rhizoma Atractylodis Macrocephalae (*Bai Zhu*), 30g, Radix Albus Paeoniae Lactiflorae (*Bai Shao*), and Radix Ledebouriellae Divaricatae (*Fang Feng*), 20g each, and Pericarpium Citri Reticulatae (*Chen Pi*), 10g. If there was constipation, stir-fried Atractylodes was changed to uncooked Atractylodes, 30g, and Fructus Perillae Frutescentis (*Zi Su Zi*), 10g, was added. If there was enduring diarrhea which would not heal, Rhizoma Cimicifugae (*Sheng Ma*), 6g, was added. One packet was administered per day, decocted in water and given orally.

The comparison group received nifepine (*Xin Tong Ding*), 10mg three times per day, and a multivitamin, 30mg, three times per day. Treatment lasted for four weeks.

Marked effect was defined as disappearance of the symptoms. Some effect meant there was a marked improvement in the symptoms. No effect meant that there was no obvious change or improvement in the symptoms. Based on these criteria, 18 cases in the treatment group got a marked effect and 10 got some effect, for a total amelioration or effectiveness rate of 84.8%. Eight cases in the comparison group got a marked effect and another six got some effect. Therefore, the total amelioration rate in the comparison group was only 58.3%. Thus there was a marked statistical difference in the outcomes between these two groups ($x2 = 5.04$, $P < 0.05$).

The authors of this article believe that, based on the main symptoms of irritable bowel syndrome of abdominal pain, distention, and diarrhea, the disease mechanisms of this disorder are liver repletion/spleen vacuity, qi mechanism depression and stagnation, and loss of regularity of the stomach and intestines. Hence, they chose to use *Tong Xie Yao Fang*, it being the main formula within the literature for this pattern.

"The Treatment of 226 Cases of Irritable Bowel Syndrome with *Jia Wei Zhu Shao Yin* (Added Flavors Atractylodes & Peony Drink)" by Shen Wen-hua & Hu Wen-lei, *Zhe Jiang Zhong Yi Za Zhi (Zhejiang Journal of Chinese Medicine)*, #3, 1998, p. 112

There were 226 patients in this study, 117 men and 109 women, ranging from 19-66 years old. The median age was 41. Their disease course had lasted 1-20 years. Eighty-eight cases were constipated, while 138 cases experienced diarrhea.

The basic formula consisted of: stir-fried Rhizoma Atractylodis Macrocephalae (*Bai Zhu*), 30g, stir-fried Radix Albus Paeoniae Lactiflorae (*Bai Shao*), Pericarpium Citri Reticulatae (*Chen Pi*), Radix Ledebouriellae Divaricatae (*Fang Feng*), Radix Linderae Strychnifoliae (*Wu Yao*), and Rhizoma Corydalis Yanhusuo (*Yan Hu Suo*), 10g each, Radix Platycodi Grandiflori (*Jie Geng*), 6g, and Rhizoma Cimicifugae (*Sheng Ma*), 5g.

If there was diarrhea, 20-30g of stir-fried Radix Astragali Membranacei (*Huang Qi*), 5g each of Fructus Evodiae Rutacarpae (*Wu Zhu Yu*) and Fructus Schizandrae Chinensis (*Wu Wei Zi*), and 10g of Fructus Pruni Mume (*Wu Mei*) were added. If there was constipation, 20g of Semen Tricosanthis Kirlowii (*Gua Luo Ren*), 10g each of Semen Pruni Armenicae (*Xing Ren*) and Semen Arecae Catechu (*Bin Lang*), and 15g of Semen Cannabis Sativae (*Huo Ma Ren*) were added. All the patients were administered this medicine for 4-8 weeks.

One hundred two cases or 45.1% were judged cured. This meant that the number of times of defecation and its accompanying symptoms were normal, and any mucus in the stools had disappeared. Likewise, any abdominal pain or distention had disappeared. After six months, there had been no recurrence. Ninety-four cases, or 41.6% got a marked effect. This meant that the number of defecations and accompanying symptoms were basically normal, mucus in the stool was markedly decreased, and any other accompanying symptoms were also markedly diminished. Thirty cases or 13.3% were improved. This meant that the numbers of their defecations and symptoms accompanying evacuations had improved, mucus had decreased, and any accompanying symptoms had also decreased. Thus, the total amelioration rate with this protocol was 100%.

The authors equate irritable bowel syndrome to the traditional Chinese medical disease categories of diarrhea and constipation, and they attribute its disease mechanisms to a combination of spleen vacuity and liver repletion. If the spleen becomes vacuous, it is easily checked or controlled by liver wood. Thus the qi mechanism becomes blocked and stagnant and upbearing and downbearing lose their normalcy. Hence there is either diarrhea or constipation.

"The Treatment of 156 Cases of Irritable Bowel Syndrome with *Yi Min Tiao Chang Tang* (Repress Irritation & Regulate the Intestines Decoction)" by Hong Zhe-ming, *Zhe Jiang Zhong Yi Za Zhi (Zhejiang Journal of Chinese Medicine)*, #3, 1998, p. 113

All 286 patients described in this article were outpatients diagnosed as suffering from irritable bowel syndrome in the digestive disease department of the Changzhou Municipal Chinese Medicine Hospital. There were 156 patients in the treatment group, 61 men and 95 women. The oldest was 61 and the youngest was 29 years old. The median age was 33.4 years. The longest disease course was 16 years and the shortest was half a year. The median duration was 4.1 years. The comparison group was comprised of 130 patients, 52 male and 78 female. The median age in this group was 33.2, while the median duration of disease was 4.1 years. Thus there was no statistical difference between these two groups in terms of their sex, age or disease duration.

The basic formula of *Yi Min Tian Chang Tang* was composed of: Radix Albus Paeoniae Lactiflorae (*Bai Shao*), Radix Sanguisorbae (*Di Yu*), and Cortex Fraxini (*Qin Pi*), 30g each, stir-fried Rhizoma Atractylodis Macrocephalae (*Bai Zhu*), Pericarpium Citri Reticulatae (*Chen Pi*), Radix Ledebouriellae Divaricatae (*Fang Feng*), Rhizoma Corydalis Yanhusuo (*Yan Hu Suo*), and Fructus Citri Aurantii (*Zhi Ke*), 10g each, and Radix Codonopsitis Pilosulae (*Dang Shen*) and Sclerotium Poriae Cocos (*Fu Ling*), 15g each.

If dampness was heavy, 10g each of Herba Agastachis Seu Pogostemi (*Huo Xiang*) and stir-fried Semen Coicis Lachryma-jobi (*Yi Yi Ren*) were added. If there was kidney yang vacuity, 10g each of Fructus Psoraleae Corylifoliae (*Bu Gu Zhi*) and roasted Fructus Myristicae Fragrantis (*Rou Dou Kou*) were added. If there was mainly diarrhea, 10g of roasted Fructus Terminaliae Chebulae (*He Zi*) and 5g of blast-fried Rhizoma Zingiberis (*Pao Jiang*) were added. If there was mainly constipation, 15g of Herba Cistanchis Deserticolae (*Rou Cong Rong*) and 5g of cooked Radix Et Rhizoma Rhei (*Da Huang*) were added. One packet was administered per day, decocted in water and divided in two portions. Two months equaled one course of treatment.

The comparison group received orally 25mg three times per day of the Western medicine doxepin and 10mg three times per day of adalat. Two months equaled one course of treatment.

Cure was defined as disappearance of the symptoms, normal defecation, normal tongue and pulse signs, disappearance of intestinal hyperemia and edema, and no recurrence after one year. Improvement was defined as basic disappearance of the symptoms, defecation essentially normal or soft stools, improvement in the tongue and pulse signs, decrease in intestinal hyperemia and edema, and no pronounced occurrence in one year. No effect meant that the symptoms and abnormalities in defecation had not improved, and/or that there were recurrences during the course of treatment.

Based on the above criteria, 62 cases in the treatment group were considered cured, 80 were improved and 14 got no effect. Thus the cure rate was 39.7% and the total amelioration rate was 91%. In the comparison group, 34 cases were cured, 57 were improved and 39 got no effect. Therefore, the cure rate in the comparison group was 26.2% and the total amelioration rate was 71.5%. Hence there was a statistically significant difference in the cure and amelioration rates between these two groups.

The author relates the cause of irritable bowel syndrome mostly to emotions, diet, and environment. In Chinese medicine, this disease is mostly due to constrained liver qi which then counterflows horizontally to assail the spleen. The spleen qi thus becomes vacuous and weak, while depressive heat, dampness, and turbidity mutually stagnate, thus resulting in this condition. If this condition endures for a long time and is not cured, enduring disease can damage the kidneys.

Lest any Western readers think that this Chinese research is less than rigorous and, therefore, to be dismissed as worthless, the prestigious *Journal of the American Medical Association* recently published an article titled "Treatment of Irritable Bowel Syndrome with Chinese Herbal Medicine" by Alan Bensoussan *et al.* In its Nov. 11, 1998 issue on pages 1585-1589. This article supports and confirms what the above Chinese clinical audits have been maintaining for decades–A) that Chinese herbal medicine can effectively treat IBS, and B) that *Tong Xie Yao Fang* is the right formula to base treatment of this condition on.

This was a prospective randomly assigned, double-blind, placebo-controlled study, supposedly the "gold standard" of modern medical research. In it, a total of 116 patients diagnosed with IBS were divided into three groups. One group of patients received a standardized Chinese herbal formula for IBS, another group received personally tailored and individualized Chinese herbal formulas from trained Chinese doctors, and the third group received a placebo. At the end of this study, patients in the two Chinese herbal groups experienced significantly more effect than did the placebo group. Although initially, patients receiving the individualized treatment got no better effect than the standardized treatment, on follow-up after 14 weeks, only those in the individualized treatment group had maintained their improvement. The standard formula used in this study was a modification of *Tong Xie Yao Fang* designed to treat as broad a spectrum of patterns as possible without "throwing in everything but the kitchen sink." It included ingredients for liver depression spleen vacuity, damp heat, and kidney qi vacuity not astringing and securing the intestines.

11 Finding a Professional Practitioner of Chinese Medicine

Traditional Chinese medicine is one of the fastest growing holistic health care systems in the West today. At the present time, there are 50 colleges in the United States alone which offer 3-4 year training programs in acupuncture, moxibustion, Chinese herbal medicine, and Chinese medical massage. In addition, many of the graduates of these programs have done postgraduate studies at colleges and hospitals in China, Taiwan, Hong Kong, and Japan. Further, a growing number of trained Oriental medical practitioners have immigrated from China, Japan, and Korea to practice acupuncture and Chinese herbal medicine in the West.

Traditional Chinese medicine, including acupuncture, is a discreet and independent health care profession. It is not simply a technique that can easily be added to the array of techniques of some other health care profession. The study of Chinese medicine, acupuncture, and Chinese herbs is as rigorous as is the study of allopathic, chiropractic, naturopathic, or homeopathic medicine. Previous training in any one of these other systems does not automatically confer competence or knowledge in Chinese medicine. In order to get the full benefits and safety of Chinese medicine, one should seek out professionally trained and credentialed practitioners.

In the United States of America, recognition that acupuncture and Chinese medicine are their own independent professions has led to the creation of the National Commission for the Certification of Acupuncture & Oriental Medicine (NCCAOM). This commission has created and administers a national board examination in both acupuncture and Chinese herbal medicine in order to insure minimum levels of professional competence and safety. Those who pass the acupuncture exam append the letters Dipl. Ac. (Diplomate of Acupuncture) after their names, while those who pass the Chinese herbal exam use the letters Dipl. C.H. (Diplomate of Chinese Herbs). I recommend that persons wishing to experience the benefits of acupuncture and Chinese medicine should seek treatment in the U.S. only from those who are NCCAOM certified.

In addition, in the United States, acupuncture is a legal, independent health care profession in more than half the states. A few other states require acupuncturists to work under the supervision of MDs, while in a number of states, acupuncture has yet to receive legal status. In states where acupuncture is licensed and regulated, the names of acupuncture practitioners can be found in the *Yellow Pages* of your local phone book or through contacting your State Department of Health, Board of Medical Examiners, or Department of Regulatory Agencies. In states without licensure, it is doubly important to seek treatment only from NCCAOM diplomates.

When seeking a qualified and knowledgeable practitioner, word of mouth referrals are important. Satisfied patients are the most reliable credential a practitioner can have. It is appropriate to ask the practitioner for references from previous patients treated for the same problem. It is best to work with a practitioner who communicates effectively enough for the patient to feel understood and for the Chinese medical diagnosis and treatment plan to make sense. In all cases, a professional practitioner of Chinese medicine should be able and willing to give a written traditional Chinese diagnosis of the patient's pattern upon request.

For further information regarding the practice of Chinese medicine and acupuncture in the United States and for referrals to local professional associations and practitioners in the United States, prospective patients may contact:

National Commission for the Certification of Acupuncture & Oriental Medicine
P.O. Box 97075
Washington DC 20090-7075
Tel: (202) 232-1404
Fax: (202) 462-6157

The National Acupuncture & Oriental Medicine Alliance
14637 Starr Rd, SE
Olalla, WA 98357
Tel: (206) 851-6895
Fax: (206) 728-4841
E mail: 76143.2061@compuserve.com

The American Association of Oriental Medicine
433 Front St.
Catasauqua, PA 18032-2506
Tel: (610) 433-2448
Fax: (610) 433-1832

12
Learning More About Chinese Medicine

For more information on Chinese medicine in general, see:

The Web That Has No Weaver: Understanding Chinese Medicine by Ted Kaptchuk, Congdon & Weed, NY, 1983. This is the best overall introduction to Chinese medicine for the serious lay reader. It has been a standard since it was first published over a dozen years ago and it has yet to be replaced.

Chinese Secrets of Health & Longevity by Bob Flaws, Sound True, Boulder, CO, 1996. This is a six tape audiocassette course introducing Chinese medicine to laypeople. It covers basic Chinese medical theory, Chinese dietary therapy, Chinese herbal medicine, acupuncture, *qi gong*, *feng shui*, deep relaxation, lifestyle, and more.

Fundamentals of Chinese Medicine by the East Asian Medical Studies Society, Paradigm Publications, Brookline, MA, 1985. This is a more technical introduction and overview of Chinese medicine intended for professional entry level students.

Traditional Medicine in Contemporary China by Nathan Sivin, Center for Chinese Studies, University of Michigan, Ann Arbor, 1987. This book discusses the development of Chinese medicine in China in the last half century as well as introducing all the basic concepts of Chinese medical theory and practice.

Rooted in Spirit: The Heart of Chinese Medicine by Claude Larre & Elisabeth Rochat de la Vallée, trans. by Sarah Stang, Station Hill Press, NY, 1995. This book explains the central concepts of Chinese medicine from a decidedly spiritual point of view. Essentially, it is commentary on the eighth chapter of the *Nei Jing Ling Shu (Inner Classic: Spiritual Pivot).*

In the Footsteps of the Yellow Emperor: Tracing the History of Traditional Acupuncture by Peter Eckman, Cypress Book Company, San Francisco, 1996. This book is a history of Chinese medicine and especially acupuncture. In it, the author traces how acupuncture came to Europe and America from China, Hong Kong, Taiwan, Japan, and Korea in the early and middle part of this century. Included are nontechnical discussions of basic Chinese medical theory and concepts.

Knowing Practice: The Clinical Encounter of Chinese Medicine by Judith Farquhar, Westview Press, Boulder, CO, 1994. This book is a more scholarly approach to the recent history of Chinese medicine in the People's Republic of China as well as an introduction to the basic methodology of Chinese medical practice. Although written by an academic sinologist and not a practitioner, it nonetheless contains many insightful and perceptive observations on the differences between traditional Chinese and modern Western medicines.

Imperial Secrets of Health and Longevity by Bob Flaws, Blue Poppy Press, Boulder, CO, 1994. This book includes a section on Chinese dietary therapy and generally introduces the basic concepts of good health according to Chinese medicine.

Chinese Herbal Remedies by Albert Y. Leung, Universe Books, NY, 1984. This book is about simple Chinese herbal home remedies.

Legendary Chinese Healing Herbs by Henry C. Lu, Sterling Publishing, Inc., NY, 1991. This book is a fun way to begin learning about Chinese herbal medicine. It is full of interesting and entertaining anecdotes about Chinese medicinal herbs.

The Mystery of Longevity by Liu Zheng-cai, Foreign Languages Press, Beijing, 1990. This book is also about general principles and practice promoting good health according to Chinese medicine.

For more information on Chinese dietary therapy, see:

The Tao of Healthy Eating According to Traditional Chinese Medicine by Bob Flaws, Blue Poppy Press, Boulder, CO, 1997. This book is a layperson's primer on Chinese dietary therapy. It includes detailed sections on the clear, bland diet as well as sections on chronic candidiasis and allergies. It also includes the Chinese medical descriptions and uses of 200 commonly eaten foods.

The Book of Jook: Chinese Medicinal Porridges, A Healthy Alternative to the Typical Western Breakfast by Bob Flaws, Blue Poppy Press, Boulder, CO, 1995. This book is specifically about Chinese medicinal porridges made with very simple combinations of Chinese medicinal herbs.

The Tao of Nutrition by Maoshing Ni, Union of Tao and Man, Los Angeles, 1989

Harmony Rules: The Chinese Way of Health Through Food by Gary Butt & Frena Bloomfield, Samuel Weiser, Inc., York Beach, ME, 1985

Chinese System of Food Cures: Prevention & Remedies by Henry C. Lu, Sterling Publishing, Inc., NY, 1986

A Practical English-Chinese Library of Traditional Chinese Medicine: Chinese Medicated Diet ed. by Zhang En-qin, Shanghai College of Traditional Chinese Medicine Publishing House, Shanghai, 1990

Eating Your Way to Health—Dietotherapy in Traditional Chinese Medicine by Cai Jing-feng, Foreign Languages Press, Beijing, 1988

Chinese Medical Glossary

Chinese medicine is a system unto itself. Its technical terms are uniquely its own and cannot be reduced to the definitions of Western medicine without destroying the very fabric and logic of Chinese medicine. Ultimately, because Chinese medicine was created in the Chinese language, Chinese medicine is best and really only understood in that language. Nevertheless, as Westerners trying to understand Chinese medicine, we must translate the technical terms of Chinese medicine in English words. If some of these technical translations sound peculiar at first and their meaning is not immediately apparent, this is because no equivalent concepts exist in everyday English.

In the past, some Western authors have erroneously translated technical Chinese medical terms using Western medical or at least quasi-scientific words in an attempt to make this system more acceptable to Western audiences. For instance, the words tonify and sedate are commonly seen in the Western Chinese medical literature even though, in the case of sedate, its meaning is 180•opposite to the Chinese understanding of the word *xie*. *Xie* means to drain off something which has pooled and accumulated. That accumulation is seen as something excess which should not be lingering where it is. Because it is accumulating somewhere where it shouldn't, it is impeding and obstructing whatever should be moving to and through that area. The word sedate comes from the Latin word *sedere*, to sit. Therefore, the word sedate means to make something sit still. In English, we get the word sediment from this same root. However, the Chinese *xie* means draining off that which is sitting somewhere erroneously. Therefore, to think that one is going to sedate what is already sitting is a great mistake in understanding the clinical implication and application of this technical term.

Therefore, in order to preserve the integrity of this system while still making it intelligible to English language readers, I have appended the following glossary of Chinese medical technical terms. The terms themselves are based on Nigel Wiseman's

English-Chinese Chinese-English Dictionary of Chinese Medicine published by the Hunan Science & Technology Press in Changsha, Hunan, People's Republic of China in 1995. Dr. Wiseman is, I believe, the greatest Western scholar in terms of the translation of Chinese medicine into English. As a Chinese reader myself, although I often find Wiseman's terms awkward sounding at first, I also think they convey most accurately the Chinese understanding and logic of these terms.

Acquired essence: Essence manufactured out of the surplus of qi and blood in turn created out of the refined essence of food and drink

Acupoints: Those places on the channels and network vessels where qi and blood tend to collect in denser concentrations, and thus those places where the qi and blood in the channels are especially available for manipulation

Acupuncture: The regulation of qi flow by the stimulation of certain points located on the channels and network vessels achieved mainly by the insertion of fine needles into these points

Aromatherapy: Using various scents and smells to treat and prevent disease

Ascendant hyperactivity of liver yang: Upwardly out of control counterflow of liver yang due to insufficient yin to hold it down in the lower part of the body

Bedroom taxation: Fatigue or vacuity due to excessive sex

Blood: The red colored fluid which flows in the vessels and nourishes and constructs the tissues of the body

Blood stasis: Also called dead blood, malign blood, and dry blood, blood stasis is blood which is no longer moving through the vessels as it should. Instead it is precipitated in the vessels like silt in a river. Like silt, it then obstructs the free flow of the blood in the vessels and also impedes the production of new or fresh blood.

Blood vacuity: Insufficient blood manifesting in diminished nourishment, construction, and moistening of body tissues

Bowels: The hollow yang organs of Chinese medicine

Central qi: Also called the middle qi, this is synonymous with the spleen-stomach qi

Channels: The main routes for the distribution of qi and blood, but mainly qi

***Chong & ren*:** Two of the eight extraordinary vessels which act as reservoirs for all the other channels and vessels of the body. These two govern women's menstruation, reproduction, and lactation in particular.

Clear: The pure or clear part of food and drink ingested which is then turned into qi and blood
Counterflow: An erroneous flow of qi, usually upward but sometimes horizontally as well
Damp heat: A combination of accumulated dampness mixed with pathological heat often associated with sores, abnormal vaginal discharges, and some types of menstrual and body pain
Dampness: A pathological accumulation of body fluids
Decoction: A method of administering Chinese medicinals by boiling these medicinals in water, removing the dregs, and drinking the resulting medicinal liquid
Depression: Stagnation and lack of movement, as in liver depression qi stagnation
Depressive heat: Heat due to enduring or severe qi stagnation which then transforms into heat
Drain: To drain off or away some pathological qi or substance from where it is replete or excess
Essence: A stored, very potent form of substance and qi, usually yin when compared to yang qi, but can be transformed into yang qi
Five phase theory: A ancient Chinese system of correspondences dividing up all of reality into five phases of development which then mutually engender and check each other according to definite sequences
Foot reflexology: The stimulation of zones on the feet which correspond with the viscera and bowels, thus a method of stimulating the internal organs by stimulating the feet.
Heat toxins: A particularly virulent and concentrated type of pathological heat often associated with purulence (*i.e.*, pus formation), sores, and sometimes, but not always, malignancies
Heliotherapy: Exposure of the body to sunlight in order to treat and prevent disease
Hydrotherapy: Using various baths and water applications to treat and prevent disease
Lassitude of the spirit: A listless or apathetic affect or emotional demeanor due to obvious fatigue of the mind and body
Life gate fire: Another name for kidney yang or kidney fire, seen as the ultimate source of yang qi in the body
Magnet therapy: Applying magnets to acupuncture points to treat and prevent disease
Moxibustion: Burning the herb Artemisia Argyium on, over, or near acupuncture points in order to add yang qi, warm cold, or promote the movement of the qi and blood

Network vessels: Small vessels which form a net-like web insuring the flow of qi and blood to all body tissues
Phlegm: A pathological accumulation of phlegm or mucus congealed from dampness or body fluids
Qi: Activity, function, that which moves, transforms, defends, restrains, and warms
Portals: Also called orifices, the openings of the sensory organs and the opening of the heart through which the spirit makes contact with the world outside
Qi mechanism: The process of transforming yin substance controlled and promoted by the qi, largely synonymous with the process of digestion
Qi vacuity: Insufficient qi manifesting in diminished movement, transformation, and function
Repletion: A state of fullness, abundance, or exuberance, almost always pathological
Seven star hammer: A small hammer with needles embedded in its head used to stimulate acupoints without actually inserting needles
Spirit: The accumulation of qi in the heart which manifests as consciousness, sensory awareness, and mental-emotional function
Stagnation: Non-movement of the qi, lack of free flow, constraint
Supplement: To add to or augment, as in supplementing the qi, blood, yin, or yang
Turbid: The yin, impure, turbid part of food and drink which is sent downward to be excreted as waste
Vacuity: Emptiness or insufficiency, typically of qi, blood, yin, or yang
Vacuity cold: Obvious signs and symptoms of cold due to a lack or insufficiency of yang qi
Vacuity heat: Heat due to hyperactive yang in turn due to insufficient controlling yin
Vessels: Main routes for distribution of qi and blood, but mainly blood
Viscera: The solid yin organs of Chinese medicine
Yin: In the body, substance and nourishment
Yin vacuity: Insufficient yin substance necessary to both nourish, control, and counterbalance yang activity
Yang: In the body, function, movement, activity, transformation
Yang vacuity: Insufficient warming and transforming function giving rise to symptoms of cold in the body

Bibliography

Chinese language sources

Cheng Dan An Zhen Jiu Xuan Ji (Cheng Dan-an's Selected Acupuncture & Moxibustion Works), ed. by Cheng Wei-fen *et al.*, Shanghai Science & Technology Press, Shanghai, 1986

Chu Zhen Zhi Liao Xue (A Study of Acupuncture Treatment), Li Zhong-yu, Sichuan Science & Technology Press, Chengdu, 1990

Dong Yuan Yi Ji (Dong-yuan's Collected Medical Works), ed. by Bao Zheng-fei *et al.*, People's Health & Hygiene Press, Beijing, 1993

Han Ying Chang Yong Yi Xue Ci Hui (Chinese-English Glossary of Commonly Used Medical Terms), Huang Xiao-kai, People's Health & Hygiene Press, Beijing, 1982

Shang Hai Lao Zhong Yi Jing Yan Xuan Bian (A Selected Compilation of Shanghai Old Doctors' Experiences), Shanghai Science & Technology Press, Shanghai, 1984

Shi Yong Zhen Jiu Tui Na Zhi Liao Xue (A Study of Practical Acupuncture, Moxibustion & Tui Na Treatments), Xia Zhi-ping, Shanghai College of Chinese Medicine Press, Shanghai, 1990

Tan Zheng Lun (Treatise on Phlegm Conditions), Hou Tian-yin & Wang Chun-hua, People's Army Press, Beijing, 1989

Yi Zong Jin Jian (The Golden Mirror of Ancestral Medicine), Wu Qian *et al.*, People's Health & Hygiene Press, Beijing, 1985

Yu Xue Zheng Zhi (Static Blood Patterns & Treatments), Zhang Xue-wen, Shanxi Science & Technology Press, Xian, 1986

Zhen Jiu Da Cheng (A Great Compendium of Acupuncture & Moxibustion), Yang Ji-zhou, People's Health & Hygiene Press, Beijing, 1983

Zhen Jiu Xue (A Study of Acupuncture & Moxibustion), Qiu Mao-liang *et al.*, Shanghai Science & Technology Press, Shanghai, 1985

Zhen Jiu Yi Xue (An Easy Study of Acupuncture & Moxibustion), Li Shou-xian, People's Health & Hygiene Press, Beijing, 1990

Zhong Guo Min Jian Cao Yao Fang (Chinese Folk Herbal Medicinal Formulas), Liu Guang-rui & Liu Shao-lin, Sichuan Science & Technology Press, Chengdu, 1992

Zhong Guo Zhen Jiu Chu Fang Xue (A Study of Chinese Acupuncture & Moxibustion Prescriptions), Xiao Shao-qing, Ningxia People's Press, Yinchuan, 1986

Zhong Guo Zhong Yi Mi Fang Da Quan (A Great Compendium of Chinese National Chinese Medical Secret Formulas), ed. by Hu Zhao-ming, Literary Propagation Publishing Company, Shanghai, 1992

Zhong Yi Hu Li Xue (A Study of Chinese Medical Nursing), Lu Su-ying, People's Health & Hygiene Press, Beijing, 1983

Zhong Yi Lin Chuang Ge Ke (Various Clinical Specialties in Chinese Medicine), Zhang En-qin *et al.*, Shanghai College of TCM Press, Shanghai, 1990

Zhong Yi Ling Yan Fang (Efficacious Chinese Medical Formulas), Lin Bin-zhi, Science & Technology Propagation Press, Beijing, 1991

Zhong Yi Zi Xue Cong Shu (The Chinese Medicine Self-study Series), Vol. 1, "Gynecology", Yang Yi-ya, Hebei Science & Technology Press, Shijiazhuang, 1987

English language sources

A Barefoot Doctor's Manual, revised & enlarged edition, Cloudburst Press, Mayne Isle, 1977

A Clinical Guide to Chinese Herbs and Formulae, Cheng Song-yu & Li Fei, Churchill & Livingstone, Edinburgh, 1993

A Compendium of TCM Patterns & Treatments, Bob Flaws & Daniel Finney, Blue Poppy Press, Boulder, CO, 1996

A Comprehensive Guide to Chinese Herbal Medicine, Chen Ze-lin & Chen Mei-fang, Oriental Healing Arts Institute, Long Beach, CA, 1992

A Handbook of Differential Diagnosis with Key Signs & Symptoms, Therapeutic Principles, and Guiding Prescriptions, Ou-yang Yi, trans. by C. S. Cheung, Harmonious Sunshine Cultural Center, San Francisco, 1987

A Manual of Acupuncture, Peter Deadman and Mazin Al-Khafaji with Kevin Baker, Journal of Chinese Medicine Publications, Hove, England, 1998

A Practical Dictionary of Chinese Medicine, second edition, Nigel Wiseman and Feng Ye, Paradigm Publications, Brookline, MA, 1998

A Practical English-Chinese Library of Traditional Chinese Medicine: Chinese Massage, Zhang Enqin, editor-in-chief, Publishing House of Shanghai College of TCM, Shanghai,1988

A Practical English-Chinese Library of Traditional Chinese Medicine: Health Preservation and Rehabilitation, Zhang Enqin, editor- in-chief, Publishing House of Shanghai College of TCM, Shanghai,1988

Arisal of the Clear: A Simple Guide to Healthy Eating According to Traditional Chinese Medicine, Bob Flaws, Blue Poppy Press, Boulder, CO, 1991

Chinese-English Terminology of Traditional Chinese Medicine, Shuai Xue-zhong *et al.*, Hunan Science & Technology Press, Changsha, 1983

Chinese-English Manual of Common-used Prescriptions in Traditional Chinese Medicine, Ou Ming, ed., Joint Publishing Co., Ltd., Hong Kong, 1989

Chinese Herbal Medicine: Formulas & Strategies, Dan Bensky & Randall Barolet, Eastland Press, Seattle, 1990

Chinese Herbal Medicine: Materia Medica, Dan Bensky & Andrew Gamble, second, revised edition, Eastland Press, Seattle, 1993

Chinese Self-massage: The Easy Way to Health, Fan Ya-li, Blue Poppy Press, Boulder, CO, 1996

Classical Moxibustion Skills, Sung Baek,, Blue Poppy Press, Boulder, CO, 1990

English-Chinese Chinese-English Dictionary of Chinese Medicine, Nigel Wiseman, Hunan Science & Technology Press, Changsha, 1995

Fundamentals of Chinese Acupuncture, Andrew Ellis, Nigel Wiseman & Ken Boss, Paradigm Publications, Brookline, MA, 1988

Fundamentals of Chinese Medicine, Nigel Wiseman & Andrew Ellis, Paradigm Publications, Brookline, MA, 1985

Glossary of Chinese Medical Terms and Acupuncture Points, Nigel Wiseman & Ken Boss, Paradigm Publications, Brookline, MA, 1990

Handbook of Chinese Herbs and Formulas, Him-che Yeung, self-published, CA, 1985

Oriental Materia Medica: A Concise Guide, Hong-yen Hsu, Oriental Healing Arts Institute, Long Beach, CA, 1986

Outline Guide to Chinese Herbal Patent Medicines in Pill Form, Margaret A. Naeser, Boston Chinese Medicine, Boston, MA, 1990

Pao Zhi: An Introduction to the Use of Processed Chinese Medicinals, Philippe Sionneau, translated by Bob Flaws, Blue Poppy Press, Boulder, CO, 1994

Practical Traditional Chinese Medicine & Pharmacology: Clinical Experiences, Shang Xian-min *et al.*, New World Press, Beijing, 1990

Practical Traditional Chinese Medicine & Pharmacology: Herbal Formulas, Geng Jun-ying, *et al.*, New World Press, Beijing, 1991

The Essential Book of Traditional Chinese Medicine, Vol. 2: Clinical Practice, Liu Yan-chi, trans. by Fang Ting-yu & Chen Lai-di, Columbia University Press, NY, 1988

The Merck Manual of Diagnosis & Therapy, 15th edition, ed. by Robert Berkow, Merck Sharp & Dohme Research Laboratories, Rahway, NJ, 1987

The Nanjing Seminars Transcript, Qiu Mao-lian & Su Xu-ming, The Journal of Chinese Medicine, UK, 1985

The Practice of Chinese Medicine: The Treatment of Diseases with Acupuncture and Chinese Herbs, Giovanni Maciocia, Churchill Livingstone, Edinburgh, 1994

The Treatise on the Spleen & Stomach, Li Dong-yuan, trans. by Yang Shou-zhong, Blue Poppy Press, Boulder, CO, 1993

The Treatment of Disease in TCM, Volume 1: Diseases of the Head and Face Including Mental/Emotional Disorders, Philippe Sionneau and Lu Gang, Blue Poppy Press, Boulder, CO, 1996

The Yeast Connection, William G. Crook, Vintage Books, Random House, NY, 1986

The Yeast Syndrome, John Parks Towbridge & Morton Walker, Bantam Books, Toronto, 1988

Traditional Medicine in Contemporary China, Nathan Sivin, University of Michigan, Ann Arbor, 1987

Zang Fu: The Organ Systems of Traditional Chinese Medicine, second edition, Jeremy Ross, Churchill Livingstone, Edinburgh, 1985

Index

E

F, G

H

I

J, L

M

N, O

P, Q

R

S

T

U, V

W, X, Y

OTHER BOOKS ON CHINESE MEDICINE AVAILABLE FROM:

BLUE POPPY PRESS

5441 Western, Suite 2, Boulder, CO 80301
For ordering 1-800-487-9296 PH. 303\447-8372 FAX 303\245-8362
Email: info@bluepoppy.com Website: www.bluepoppy.com

ACUPOINT POCKET REFERENCE by Bob Flaws
ISBN 0-936185-93-7
ISBN 978-0-936185-93-4

ACUPUNCTURE & IVF by Lifang Liang
ISBN 0-891845-24-1
ISBN 978-0-891845-24-6

ACUPUNCTURE FOR STROKE REHABILITATION
Three Decades of Information from China
by Hoy Ping Yee Chan, *et al.*
ISBN 1-891845-35-7
ISBN 978-1-891845-35-2

ACUPUNCTURE PHYSICAL MEDICINE: An Acupuncture Touchpoint Approach to the Treatment of Chronic Pain, Fatigue, and Stress Disorders
by Mark Seem
ISBN 1-891845-13-6
ISBN 978-1-891845-13-0

AGING & BLOOD STASIS: A New Approach to TCM Geriatrics by Yan De-xin
ISBN 0-936185-63-6
ISBN 978-0-936185-63-7

A NEW AMERICAN ACUPUNTURE By Mark Seem
ISBN 0-936185-44-9
ISBN 978-0-936185-44-6

BETTER BREAST HEALTH NATURALLY with CHINESE MEDICINE
by Honora Lee Wolfe & Bob Flaws
ISBN 0-936185-90-2
ISBN 978-0-936185-90-3

BIOMEDICINE: A Textbook for Practitioners of Acupuncture and Oriental Medicine
by Bruce H. Robinson, MD
ISBN 1-891845-38-1
ISBN 978-1-891845-38-3

THE BOOK OF JOOK:
Chinese Medicinal Porridges
by B. Flaws
ISBN 0-936185-60-6
ISBN 978-0-936185-60-0

CHANNEL DIVERGENCES
Deeper Pathways of the Web
by Miki Shima and Charles Chase
ISBN 1-891845-15-2
ISBN 978-1-891845-15-4

CHINESE MEDICAL OBSTETRICS
by Bob Flaws
ISBN 1-891845-30-6
ISBN 978-1-891845-30-7

CHINESE MEDICAL PALMISTRY:
Your Health in Your Hand
by Zong Xiao-fan & Gary Liscum
ISBN 0-936185-64-3
ISBN 978-0-936185-64-4

CHINESE MEDICAL PSYCHIATRY
A Textbook and Clinical Manual
by Bob Flaws and James Lake, MD
ISBN 1-845891-17-9
ISBN 978-1-845891-17-8

CHINESE MEDICINAL TEAS: Simple, Proven, Folk Formulas for Common Diseases & Promoting Health
by Zong Xiao-fan & Gary Liscum
ISBN 0-936185-76-7
ISBN 978-0-936185-76-7

CHINESE MEDICINAL WINES & ELIXIRS
by Bob Flaws
ISBN 0-936185-58-9
ISBN 978-0-936185-58-3

CHINESE MEDICINE & HEALTHY WEIGHT MANAGEMENT: An Evidence-based Integrated Approach by Juliette Aiyana, L. Ac.
ISBN 1-891845-44-6
ISBN 978-1-891845-44-4

CHINESE PEDIATRIC MASSAGE THERAPY: A Parent's & Practitioner's Guide to the Prevention & Treatment of Childhood Illness
by Fan Ya-li
ISBN 0-936185-54-6
ISBN 978-0-936185-54-5

CHINESE SELF-MASSAGE THERAPY:
The Easy Way to Health
by Fan Ya-li
ISBN 0-936185-74-0
ISBN 978-0-936185-74-3

THE CLASSIC OF DIFFICULTIES:
A Translation of the Nan Jing
translation by Bob Flaws
ISBN 1-891845-07-1
ISBN 978-1-891845-07-9

A COMPENDIUM OF CHINESE MEDICAL MENSTRUAL DISEASES
by Bob Flaws
ISBN 1-891845-31-4
ISBN 978-1-891845-31-4

CONTROLLING DIABETES NATURALLY WITH CHINESE MEDICINE
by Lynn Kuchinski
ISBN 0-936185-06-3
ISBN 978-0-936185-06-2

CURING ARTHRITIS NATURALLY WITH CHINESE MEDICINE
by Douglas Frank & Bob Flaws
ISBN 0-936185-87-2
ISBN 978-0-936185-87-3

CURING DEPRESSION NATURALLY WITH CHINESE MEDICINE
by Rosa Schnyer & Bob Flaws
ISBN 0-936185-94-5
ISBN 978-0-936185-94-1

CURING FIBROMYALGIA NATURALLY WITH CHINESE MEDICINE
by Bob Flaws
ISBN 1-891845-09-8
ISBN 978-1-891845-09-3

CURING HAY FEVER NATURALLY WITH CHINESE MEDICINE
by Bob Flaws
ISBN 0-936185-91-0
ISBN 978-0-936185-91-0

CURING HEADACHES NATURALLY WITH CHINESE MEDICINE
by Bob Flaws
ISBN 0-936185-95-3
ISBN 978-0-936185-95-8

CURING IBS NATURALLY WITH CHINESE MEDICINE
by Jane Bean Oberski
ISBN 1-891845-11-X
ISBN 978-1-891845-11-6

CURING INSOMNIA NATURALLY WITH CHINESE MEDICINE
by Bob Flaws
ISBN 0-936185-86-4
ISBN 978-0-936185-86-6

CURING PMS NATURALLY WITH CHINESE MEDICINE
by Bob Flaws
ISBN 0-936185-85-6
ISBN 978-0-936185-85-9

DISEASES OF THE KIDNEY & BLADDER
by Hoy Ping Yee Chan, *et al.*
ISBN 1-891845-37-3
ISBN 978-1-891845-35-6

THE DIVINE FARMER'S MATERIA MEDICA
A Translation of the Shen Nong Ben Cao
translation by Yang Shouz-zhong
ISBN 0-936185-96-1
ISBN 978-0-936185-96-5

DUI YAO: THE ART OF COMBINING CHINESE HERBAL MEDICINALS
by Philippe Sionneau
ISBN 0-936185-81-3
ISBN 978-0-936185-81-1

ENDOMETRIOSIS, INFERTILITY AND TRADITIONAL CHINESE MEDICINE:
A Laywoman's Guide
by Bob Flaws
ISBN 0-936185-14-7
ISBN 978-0-936185-14-9

THE ESSENCE OF LIU FENG-WU'S GYNECOLOGY
by Liu Feng-wu, translated by Yang Shou-zhong
ISBN 0-936185-88-0
ISBN 978-0-936185-88-0

EXTRA TREATISES BASED ON INVESTIGATION & INQUIRY:
A Translation of Zhu Dan-xi's Ge Zhi Yu Lun
translation by Yang Shou-zhong
ISBN 0-936185-53-8
ISBN 978-0-936185-53-8

FIRE IN THE VALLEY: TCM Diagnosis & Treatment of Vaginal Diseases
by Bob Flaws
ISBN 0-936185-25-2
ISBN 978-0-936185-25-5

FU QING-ZHU'S GYNECOLOGY
trans. by Yang Shou-zhong and Liu Da-wei
ISBN 0-936185-35-X
ISBN 978-0-936185-35-4

FULFILLING THE ESSENCE:
A Handbook of Traditional & Contemporary Treatments for Female Infertility
by Bob Flaws
ISBN 0-936185-48-1
ISBN 978-0-936185-48-4

GOLDEN NEEDLE WANG LE-TING: A 20th Century Master's Approach to Acupuncture
by Yu Hui-chan and Han Fu-ru, trans. by Shuai Xue-zhong
ISBN 0-936185-78-3
ISBN 978-0-936185-78-1

A HANDBOOK OF TCM PATTERNS & THEIR TREATMENTS
by Bob Flaws & Daniel Finney
ISBN 0-936185-70-8
ISBN 978-0-936185-70-5

A HANDBOOK OF TRADITIONAL CHINESE DERMATOLOGY
by Liang Jian-hui, trans. by Zhang Ting-liang & Bob Flaws
ISBN 0-936185-46-5
ISBN 978-0-936185-46-0

A HANDBOOK OF TRADITIONAL CHINESE GYNECOLOGY
by Zhejiang College of TCM, trans. by Zhang Ting-liang & Bob Flaws
ISBN 0-936185-06-6 (4th edit.)
ISBN 978-0-936185-06-4

A HANDBOOK OF CHINESE HEMATOLOGY
by Simon Becker
ISBN 1-891845-16-0
ISBN 978-1-891845-16-1

A HANDBOOK of TCM PEDIATRICS
by Bob Flaws
ISBN 0-936185-72-4
ISBN 978-0-936185-72-9

THE HEART & ESSENCE OF DAN-XI'S METHODS OF TREATMENT
by Xu Dan-xi, trans. by Yang Shou-zhong
ISBN 0-926185-50-3
ISBN 978-0-936185-50-7

HERB TOXICITIES & DRUG INTERACTIONS:
A Formula Approach by Fred Jennes with Bob Flaws
ISBN 1-891845-26-8
ISBN 978-1-891845-26-0

IMPERIAL SECRETS OF HEALTH & LONGEVITY
by Bob Flaws
ISBN 0-936185-51-1
ISBN 978-0-936185-51-4

INSIGHTS OF A SENIOR ACUPUNCTURIST
by Miriam Lee
ISBN 0-936185-33-3
ISBN 978-0-936185-33-0

INTEGRATED PHARMACOLOGY: Combining Modern Pharmacology with Chinese Medicine
by Dr. Greg Sperber with Bob Flaws
ISBN 1-891845-41-1
ISBN 978-0-936185-41-3

INTRODUCTION TO THE USE OF PROCESSED CHINESE MEDICINALS
by Philippe Sionneau
ISBN 0-936185-62-7
ISBN 978-0-936185-62-0

KEEPING YOUR CHILD HEALTHY WITH CHINESE MEDICINE
by Bob Flaws
ISBN 0-936185-71-6
ISBN 978-0-936185-71-2

THE LAKESIDE MASTER'S STUDY OF THE PULSE
by Li Shi-zhen, trans. by Bob Flaws
ISBN 1-891845-01-2
ISBN 978-1-891845-01-7

MANAGING MENOPAUSE NATURALLY WITH CHINESE MEDICINE
by Honora Lee Wolfe
ISBN 0-936185-98-8
ISBN 978-0-936185-98-9

MASTER HUA'S CLASSIC OF THE CENTRAL VISCERA
by Hua Tuo, trans. by Yang Shou-zhong
ISBN 0-936185-43-0
ISBN 978-0-936185-43-9

THE MEDICAL I CHING: Oracle of the Healer Within
by Miki Shima
ISBN 0-936185-38-4
ISBN 978-0-936185-38-5

MENOPAIUSE & CHINESE MEDICINE
by Bob Flaws
ISBN 1-891845-40-3
ISBN 978-1-891845-40-6

MOXIBUSTION: The Power of Mugwort Fire
by Lorraine Wilcox
ISBN 1-891845-46-2
ISBN 978-1-891845-46-8

TEST PREP WORKBOOK FOR THE NCCAOM BIO-MEDICINE MODULE: Exam Preparation & Study Guide
by Zhong Bai-song
ISBN 1-891845-34-9
ISBN 978-1-891845-34-5

POINTS FOR PROFIT: The Essential Guide to Practice Success for Acupuncturists 3rd Edition
by Honora Wolfe, Eric Strand & Marilyn Allen
ISBN 1-891845-25-X
ISBN 978-1-891845-25-3

PRINCIPLES OF CHINESE MEDICAL ANDROLOGY: An Integrated Approach to Male Reproductive and Urological Health by Bob Damone
ISBN 1-891845-45-4
ISBN 978-1-891845-45-1

PRINCE WEN HUI's COOK: Chinese Dietary Therapy
By Bob Flaws & Honora Wolfe
ISBN 0-912111-05-4
ISBN 978-0-912111-05-6

THE PULSE CLASSIC: A Translation of the Mai Jing
by Wang Shu-he, trans. by Yang Shou-zhong
ISBN 0-936185-75-9
ISBN 978-0-936185-75-0

THE SECRET OF CHINESE PULSE DIAGNOSIS
by Bob Flaws
ISBN 0-936185-67-8
ISBN 978-0-936185-67-5

SECRET SHAOLIN FORMULAS for the Treatment of External Injury
by De Chan, trans. by Zhang Ting-liang & Bob Flaws
ISBN 0-936185-08-2
ISBN 978-0-936185-08-8

STATEMENTS OF FACT IN TRADITIONAL CHINESE MEDICINE Revised & Expanded
by Bob Flaws
ISBN 0-936185-52-X
ISBN 978-0-936185-52-1

STICKING TO THE POINT 1: A Rational Methodology for the Step by Step Formulation & Administration of an Acupuncture Treatment
by Bob Flaws
ISBN 0-936185-17-1
ISBN 978-0-936185-17-0

STICKING TO THE POINT 2: A Study of Acupuncture & Moxibustion Formulas and Strategies
by Bob Flaws
ISBN 0-936185-97-X
ISBN 978-0-936185-97-2

A STUDY OF DAOIST ACUPUNCTURE & MOXIBUSTION
by Liu Zheng-cai
ISBN 1-891845-08-X
ISBN 978-1-891845-08-6

THE SUCCESSFUL CHINESE HERBALIST
by Bob Flaws and Honora Lee Wolfe
ISBN 1-891845-29-2
ISBN 978-1-891845-29-1

THE SYSTEMATIC CLASSIC OF ACUPUNCTURE & MOXIBUSTION
A translation of the Jia Yi Jing
by Huang-fu Mi, trans. by Yang Shou-zhong & Charles Chace
ISBN 0-936185-29-5
ISBN 978-0-936185-29-3

THE TAO OF HEALTHY EATING ACCORDING TO CHINESE MEDICINE
by Bob Flaws
ISBN 0-936185-92-9
ISBN 978-0-936185-92-7

TEACH YOURSELF TO READ MODERN MEDICAL CHINESE
by Bob Flaws
ISBN 0-936185-99-6
ISBN 978-0-936185-99-6

TEST PREP WORKBOOK FOR BASIC TCM THEORY
by Zhong Bai-song
ISBN 1-891845-43-8
ISBN 978-1-891845-43-7

TREATING PEDIATRIC BED-WETTING WITH ACUPUNCTURE & CHINESE MEDICINE
by Robert Helmer
ISBN 1-891845-33-0
ISBN 978-1-891845-33-8

TREATISE on the SPLEEN & STOMACH: A Translation and annotation of Li Dong-yuan's *Pi Wei Lun*
by Bob Flaws
ISBN 0-936185-41-4
ISBN 978-0-936185-41-5

THE TREATMENT OF CARDIOVASCULAR DISEASES WITH CHINESE MEDICINE
by Simon Becker, Bob Flaws & Robert Casañas, MD
ISBN 1-891845-27-6
ISBN 978-1-891845-27-7

THE TREATMENT OF DIABETES MELLITUS WITH CHINESE MEDICINE
by Bob Flaws, Lynn Kuchinski & Robert Casañas, M.D.
ISBN 1-891845-21-7
ISBN 978-1-891845-21-5

THE TREATMENT OF DISEASE IN TCM, Vol. 1: Diseases of the Head & Face, Including Mental & Emotional Disorders
by Philippe Sionneau & Lü Gang
ISBN 0-936185-69-4
ISBN 978-0-936185-69-9

THE TREATMENT OF DISEASE IN TCM, Vol. II: Diseases of the Eyes, Ears, Nose, & Throat
by Sionneau & Lü
ISBN 0-936185-73-2
ISBN 978-0-936185-73-6

THE TREATMENT OF DISEASE IN TCM, Vol. III: Diseases of the Mouth, Lips, Tongue, Teeth & Gums
by Sionneau & Lü
ISBN 0-936185-79-1
ISBN 978-0-936185-79-8

THE TREATMENT OF DISEASE IN TCM, Vol IV: Diseases of the Neck, Shoulders, Back, & Limbs
by Philippe Sionneau & Lü Gang
ISBN 0-936185-89-9
ISBN 978-0-936185-89-7

THE TREATMENT OF DISEASE IN TCM, Vol V: Diseases of the Chest & Abdomen
by Philippe Sionneau & Lü Gang
ISBN 1-891845-02-0
ISBN 978-1-891845-02-4

THE TREATMENT OF DISEASE IN TCM, Vol VI: Diseases of the Urogential System & Proctology
by Philippe Sionneau & Lü Gang
ISBN 1-891845-05-5
ISBN 978-1-891845-05-5

THE TREATMENT OF DISEASE IN TCM, Vol VII: General Symptoms
by Philippe Sionneau & Lü Gang
ISBN 1-891845-14-4
ISBN 978-1-891845-14-7

THE TREATMENT OF EXTERNAL DISEASES WITH ACUPUNCTURE & MOXIBUSTION
by Yan Cui-lan and Zhu Yun-long, trans. by Yang Shou-zhong
ISBN 0-936185-80-5
ISBN 978-0-936185-80-4

THE TREATMENT OF MODERN WESTERN MEDICAL DISEASES WITH CHINESE MEDICINE
by Bob Flaws & Philippe Sionneau
ISBN 1-891845-20-9
ISBN 978-1-891845-20-8

UNDERSTANDING THE DIFFICULT PATIENT: A Guide for Practitioners of Oriental Medicine
by Nancy Bilello, RN, L.ac.
ISBN 1-891845-32-2
ISBN 978-1-891845-32-1

YI LIN GAI CUO (Correcting the Errors in the Forest of Medicine)
by Wang Qing-ren
ISBN 1-891845-39-X
ISBN 978-1-891845-39-0

70 ESSENTIAL CHINESE HERBAL FORMULAS
by Bob Flaws
ISBN 0-936185-59-7
ISBN 978-0-936185-59-0

160 ESSENTIAL CHINESE READY-MADE MEDICINES
by Bob Flaws
ISBN 1-891945-12-8
ISBN 978-1-891945-12-3

630 QUESTIONS & ANSWERS ABOUT CHINESE HERBAL MEDICINE: A Workbook & Study Guide
by Bob Flaws
ISBN 1-891845-04-7
ISBN 978-1-891845-04-8

260 ESSENTIAL CHINESE MEDICINALS
by Bob Flaws
ISBN 1-891845-03-9
ISBN 978-1-891845-03-1

750 QUESTIONS & ANSWERS ABOUT ACUPUNCTURE Exam Preparation & Study Guide
by Fred Jennes
ISBN 1-891845-22-5
ISBN 978-1-891845-22-2